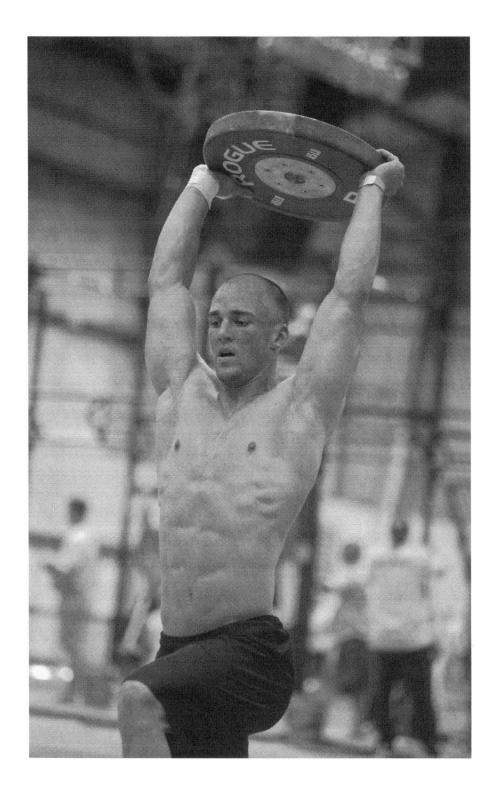

TRAINING FOR THE CROSSFIT GAMES

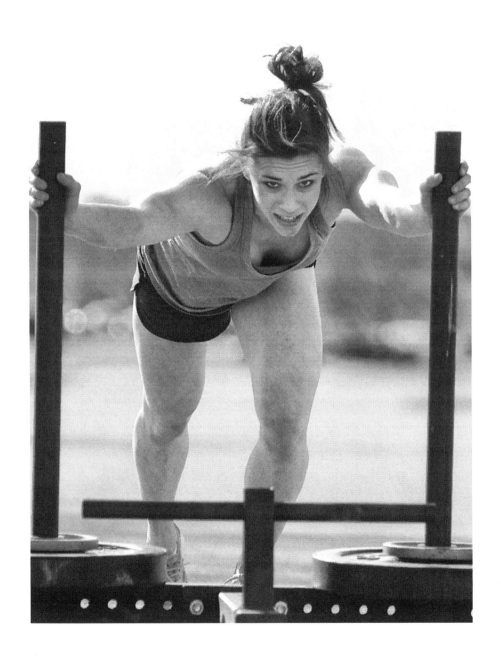

Training for the CrossFit Games

A YEAR OF PROGRAMMING
USED TO TRAIN JULIE FOUCHER,
THE 2ND FITTEST WOMAN ON EARTH,
CROSSFIT GAMES 2012

BY CROSSFIT ANN ARBOR COACH
DOUG CHAPMAN

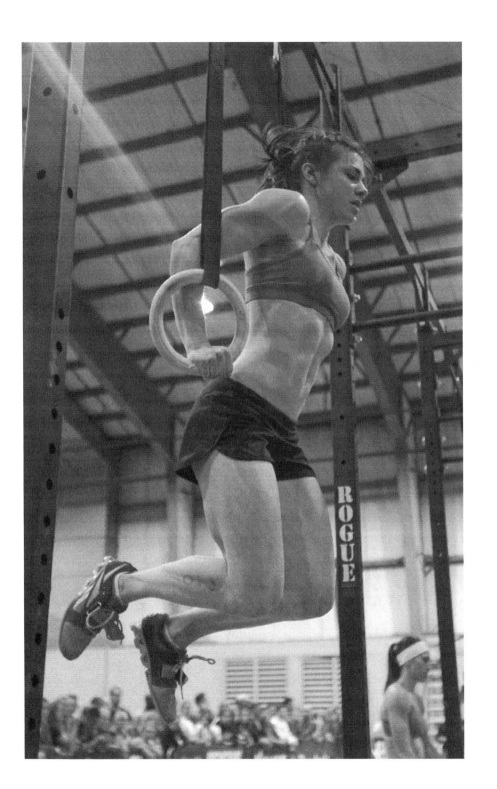

MEDICAL DISCLAIMER

The exercises described in this book may (and probably will) cause serious injury or death, especially when attempted by participants in ill or precarious health, or those who function at less than the required level of strength, endurance, and agility; or when performed using less than correct form.

In any case, consult your physician before following this (or any) exercise regimen; also, professional supervision by an experienced, CrossFit-certified trainer is highly recommended. The reader is encouraged to modify any and all exercises described herein, to fit one's particular physical condition, so as to minimize the risk of injury and to maintain the highest level of safety.

The authors and publishers hereby disclaim any and all liability for any injuries sustained while attempting, or any conditions arising (directly or indirectly) from the performance of, any exercises or training programs described in this book.

Published by HyperFit System, Inc.
Cover photography by Doug Chapman.
Interior photography by Kimberly Potterf.
CrossFit is a registered trademark of CrossFit, Inc.

Tickled Planet Publishing:
Cover design and visuals by Douglas Homer.
Product development by Julia Benben.
Editing and arrangement by Boris Shubin.

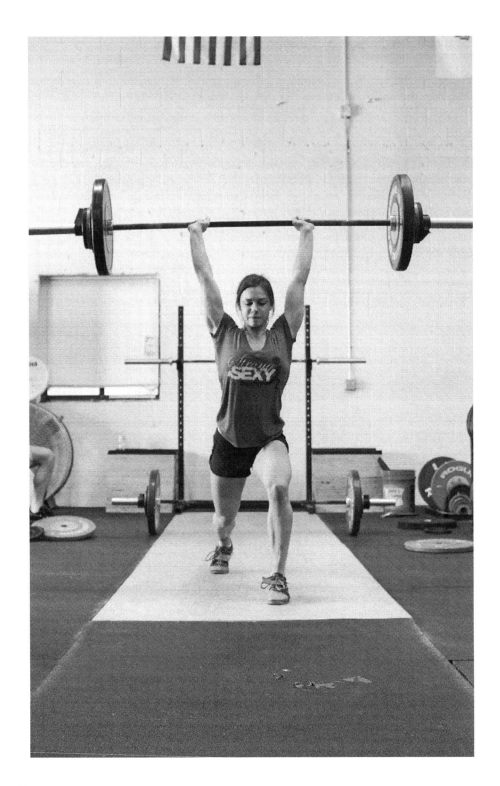

Foreword

2009-2010 Season

It was spring of 2009 that I first caught wind of CrossFit; shortly after that, I contacted Doug about completing an introductory session. A few days later, I got on my bike and rode three miles from the University of Michigan campus to HyperFit USA. I walked into the gym, and as soon as Doug introduced himself to me and shook my hand, I knew I had found my new home. I had desperately missed the environment where I grew up as a gymnast; as I looked out at the gym floor complete with pull-up rig, barbells, and a balance beam, I could hardly contain my excitement. The similarities between Doug and my childhood gymnastics coaches were immediately apparent, and allowed me to place complete trust in him as a trainer and coach.

As I progressed through my first month of one-on-one sessions, and later joined group classes, it was clear that I had a long way to go. With seemingly nothing to lose, I committed to training for competition with a small group of HyperFit USA members in early September 2009. With hardly any previous weightlifting experience, and a recent training regimen consisting of only long, slow endurance exercise, my strength was seriously lacking. I can still remember my first 100# clean and jerk that fall. My form broke down, and it felt like I was lifting the world. I never would have guessed that in a year's time, I would be lifting 155# above my head. In those early days a 200# deadlift was a serious accomplishment; a PR that would soon be shattered by a 285# lift in the 2010 Central East Regional competition. That fall consisted almost exclusively of building strength, with my beloved metcons few and far between. I was often frustrated with my slow progress during this period. It seemed that everyone around me was making large gains, and I was stuck in place.

Keeping my faith in Doug's programming, I diligently followed the plans laid out for me each day, and gave each task my best effort. As the metcon frequency and volume of training began to increase around January 2010, I started to see the previous months' labor come to fruition. Each time I performed a benchmark workout, I would PR not by seconds but minutes. By the time Regionals rolled around in May, I had posted a Fran time of 3:33 (down from 4:58 in my first Rx attempt), a Grace time of 2:20 (down from 5:18), and a FGB score of 320 (up from 268).

The gains I made in the 2 months between Regionals and the 2010 CrossFit Games were equally astonishing, as I posted a 3:14 Fran, a 2:06 Grace, and a 369 FGB.

I share these numbers to demonstrate the power of Doug's programming and coaching. In less than a year's time, I progressed from a relatively weak athlete just trying to navigate a barbell, and decipher the difference between a press and a push jerk, to finishing in 5th place at the CrossFit Games. I attribute this success to the programming in this book, combined with Doug's coaching and attention to proper movement. Doug has a way of knowing how to push you just to the point of breaking - believe me, I was there many times during this year, and it was not fun. Trusting that there was a method to the madness, and committing to never waver from his programming, I was amazed by the adaptations I witnessed in my body (and mind) over this short time.

2010-2011 Season

After seeing such dramatic improvements over the course of the 2009-2010 season, I expected a slower rate ofprogress in 2010-2011. Boy, was I wrong! Looking back, I think the 2010-2011 season marks the year of greatest improvement for me in my time as a CrossFit Games competitor.

In January 2011, Doug began to implement skill sets into the programming, from dead-hang pull-ups, dips, and muscleups, to L-sits, rope climbs, and heavy kettlebell swings. I saw dramatic improvements in my strength after just a couple of weeks. This strength and skill base was a foundation for further development, with metcons and more specific skill work later in the year. A significant amount of time (about ninety minutes, twice a week) was also dedicated to Olympic weightlifting for much of this training season. This investment really paid off, as my snatch PR increased from 120# to 150#, and my clean and jerk PR from 155# to 180#, over the course of the year. Gross conditioning, in the form ofbutcher pushes and sled pulls, also contributed to my gross strength base.

Again this year, committing diligently to Doug's programming allowed me to experience countless improvements: a 2:29 Fran (down from 3:14), over 28 rounds of Cindy (up from 22), and a 1:50 Grace time (down from 2:20). I was excited to see the adaptations of my body to this training program, and how each of the workouts and skills that Doug programs fit into a larger picture. I learned that small, deliberate, daily efforts add up over time; they are essential to success under stress. I am confident that it was the faith I had in Doug's programming, and the patience I learned while carrying it out,that contributed to such dramatic improvements this year.

2011-2012 Season - The actual programming in this book!

The 2011-2012 CrossFit Games season was a year of transition, as I moved out of state, and started a new chapter of my life as a medical student. These changes also forced me to say goodbye to HyperFit USA, and settle for a longdistance relationship with my coach. In the midst of all of these changes and uncertainties, my training (and specifically Doug's programming) was the one constant I could always count on. I knew that each week, I would receive a WOD plan with all of my tasks clearly spelled out, and that by completing each of these daily tasks, I would continue to improve.

The year began with a series of lifting cycles, each week rotating between sets of 5, 3, or 1 of the major lifts. After a few PR lifts early in the season, I hit a plateau, and became quite frustrated by my apparent lack of progress. As in previous years, however, the work started to pay off, and my numbers improved as the season continued. A number of changes were implemented this season, and several old favorites returned. Continued attention to gymnastics skills, heavy kettlebell swings, and gross conditioning such as sled pulls, butcher pushes, and farmer's walks provided me with a strong base throughout the year.

New this year was an emphasis on training camps, instead of local competitions. I liked this approach better. It allowed me to maximize my time at home during breaks from school, with large volumes of training in addition to spending time with other athletes. The 2011-2012 season also marked the debut of Doug's "MoFo" training plan. I didn't think it was possible to simultaneously love and hate something to quite the degree that I felt about this training. Doug used this program between the 2012 Regionals and Games, and I don't think anything could have prepared me more effectively for competition. Lifting near-maximal loads with brief periods of rest mimicked what I would be asked to do at the CrossFit Games, and allowed me to make tremendous gains mentally and physically in this short time.

Overall, this year again saw a great deal of improvement in many of my lifts and benchmark workouts, as I added 15# to my back squat, 10# to my clean and jerk, and achieved milestones such as a 200# overhead squat and split jerk, a 300# deadlift, a 1:39 Grace, a 2:36 Diane, and a sub-20 Kelly. More importantly, I saw significant improvement in my 3-rep, 5-rep, and 7-rep lifts, and also in my mental approach to training and competition.

In a time of transition, under the demands of medical school, I refused to waiver from the source of consistency that is Doug's programming and coaching. Perseverance paved the way to my success, and finally to a podium finish at the CrossFit Games 2012. The comprehensiveness and consistency of this training plan undoubtedly make participants fitter and more prepared for competition.

Whether you are a beginner, seasoned CrossFit athlete, or coach, I am confident that you will find the programming laid out in this book informative and beneficial. I hope that drawing from Doug's expertise and experience will enrich your own understanding of programming for the CrossFit Games, and that you may incorporate some of his ideas into your own training plan. However you choose to use this material, my best advice as an athlete is to find or develop a comprehensive training plan, and stick to it. Trust in the programming, train hard, and good luck!

Julie Foucher - Second Fittest Woman on Earth, CrossFit Games 2012 (2nd place).

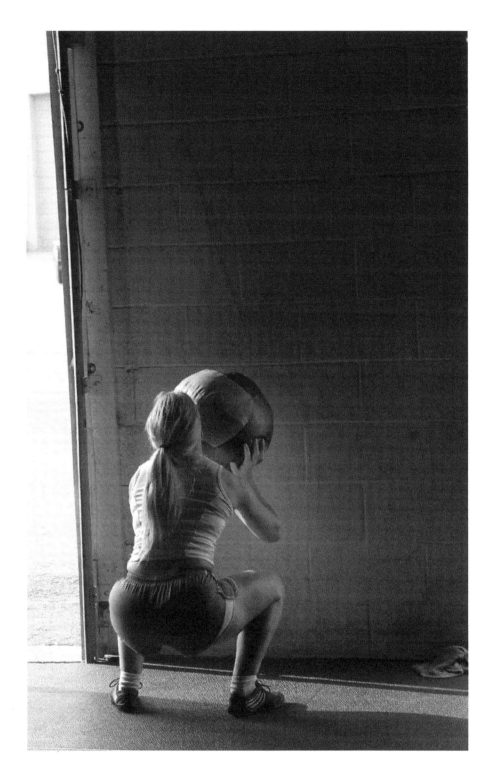

Introduction

Thank you for buying this book.

WHAT IT IS:
It is training that was programmed from the end of the CrossFit Games in 2011, through to the CrossFit Games of 2012. The programming sought to increase overall capacity in just about anything that could be tested in the CrossFit Games. The methodology is geared to minimizing weaknesses, by consistent and frequent exposure to varied skill sets. It is an amalgam of nine years of programming experience at HyperFit USA (CrossFit Ann Arbor). It is the sum total of training experience. It is a snapshot of what we did.

It is an opinion expressed in blood and sweat. It is an opinion of what it takes to make top-level Games competitors. Opinions should be based on reason, science and observation. The programming is just that.

It is the real-world application of training knowledge, geared toward producing the best generalist. There are many really great theories about developing athletes for various sports with varied time domains and skill demands. There are training systems focused on powerlifting, Olympic weightlifting, sprinting, distance running, strongman and gymnastics. All of them, and none of them, apply to our goals. All contain ideas that have some elasticity of transference, for our purposes. The training we did was based on our perspective.

The purposes of this book are several. Primarily, it is the training we used to prepare our people for the highest expression of fitness there is, the CrossFit Games. It is also a record of how we operated our gym. We do not separate our aspiring Games athletes from our base program. We believe that at its core, CrossFit is a general physical preparedness program, broadening and deepening the human capability to do work in many testable areas. Having our best people work alongside our newest people underlies one of the key tenets of CrossFit: that it is infinitely scaleable.

WHAT IT IS NOT:
It is not what you should do. The intended use of this book is as a guide and idea generator for your training. The reader may not have (and the book does not provide) the years of development that precede this snapshot. It is very difficult to just jump into the training.

It is not a look-at-me or how-cool-are-we. That is what Facebook and Twitter are for.

There are as many opinions as there are coaches. We are not a bunch of drama queens who thrive on attention. The intention of this book is to help the entire community.

It is not what we are currently using for training. Coaching and programming develop over time. There were many great lessons learned from the 2012 Games season. Many of them are being used now, with further tweaks and changes.

It is not a technique guide. Proper technique is beyond the scope of the book. If you record a video of yourself, and your form is close to the very best CrossFit form, that's great. If you look like a monkey humping a football, please slow down, learn to move correctly, and then try some of the programming. The volume presented here requires optimal technique.

GETTING THE MOST OUT OF THE BOOK:
This is a day-by-day training history of what we did, in a year of programming. There are examples of what can be done, what to do and what to avoid. Only the discerning reader will know the difference.

If I started an affiliate today, I would use this book as an idea guide on packaging and delivering the training experience.It is an excellent starting point. There are ideas for dynamic warm-up in a large class; ideas for equipment requirements for running classes; yet other ideas for integrating strength training to support basic programming.

IF YOU ARE NEW TO CROSSFIT:
This can give you good insight into what Games-level training looks like. If you are not a CrossFit practitioner, then please do not just jump in and attempt these workouts, without detailed knowledge of each movement (specifically as practiced within the CrossFit methodology). It is helpful to join the local affiliate and take some foundations classes, and learn proper form, in order to perform these movements safely. Each of these moves can be scaled to work at all levels, as we did for many members at HyperFit USA (CrossFit Ann Arbor).

One of the best sources of knowledge is www.crossfit.com.

As of this date (March 2013), there is a great FAQ section at:
http://www.crossfit.com/cf-info/faq.html
Additionally, you can see videos and explanations of movements at:
http://www.crossfit.com/cf-info/excercise.html (note: that is not a typo).

ADDITIONAL NOTES ON THE CONTENT:
Here are a few more useful thoughts regarding the philosophy, the system, and the purpose of publishing what we programmed as training for the 2012 Games. This material is not a rigid recipe, usable only and exactly in the way it is presented here. Some athletes do all of the training, in sequence, to the end. Some perform the program by segments, alternating with recovery. All practitioners will use the HyperFit System in ways that seem best suited to their individual needs and schedules.

Sometimes, circumstances disrupt the training schedule. Good judgement is critical to applying this methodology successfully, within the framework of everyday life. A level of volume or intensity that is higher than an individual's maximum capacity at a given time, can (and likely, will) result in injury.

CAUTION: The total setup for programming, as presented here, can be considered "high volume." To be prepared for a multi-day, multi-modality competition, athletes need to be able to handle an unpredictable quantity and variety of events. I think of volume a little differently. Weightlifting reps are only counted when they are over 80% of one-rep maximum. Total METCON volume is measured in terms of total time at 90%+ intensity. Volume is calculated in terms of total time at intensity and total reps over 80% each week. An individual's performance thus provides metrics for deriving volume.

One common (and critical) issue for athletes is improper form (or basic sequencing problems). Some are uncommonly gifted, and are good competitors regardless of how they move. They are few and rare, and are still very likely to experience soreness and suboptimal condition due to poor technique. A lack of attention to detail on basic movements can cause joint pain far greater than the recovery symptoms normal in fitness practitioners. To successfully attempt a program of this intensity, it is vital to move properly. It is not enough to believe one's form is correct; in order to withstand the demands of the system, one's technique actually has to be proper. If this is not the case, one must ignore the ego, drop weight, and retrain poor movement patterns to the required standard. Many initial strength gains come with correct form. I can not emphasize this enough: PROPER TECHNIQUE IS CRUCIAL.

The daily chapters contain different sections. The first section covers the classes we did in our box, and in other affiliates. These classes have some common components. The training usually includes a warm-up; some are general, and others are multifaceted and dynamic. The next component is either a WOD or Max Effort training. The sequence of these two items also changes at times, true to the ideal that CrossFit should be constantly varied. The classes often include extensive skills sets and movement progressions to help people move better. There may be notes to indicate if people on the games track should take a rest day, or complete all or some of what is programmed on that day. The programming is built around a highly organized, instructor-led training session. Each affiliate is different: some are more structured, some less. I have a tightly regimented training and instruction program; that doesn't make it right for everyone.

Each class lasts an hour. If the WOD seems short, consider a longer skill set. We sometimes budget time for people to work on skills during class, or after class. Skill sets are intended to develop movement patterns. In HyperFit programming methodology, they are targeted to minimize weakness and maintain strengths. Athletes can also use these skill sets as periods of recovery for other, higher-intensity sections of training.

When something is programmed as strict, it means kipping is not appropriate.

Much of the lifting we do is on the minute, or every three minutes, depending on the time of year and explicit goals. I believe this approach provides a well-organized class.

MoFo: This is a variation I created to get the maximum density of training. The structure is pretty simple, and therefore very tough. Athletes will need to establish 1RM for these lifts. The movements are paired; for example, M1 and M2 (meaning, Movement 1 and Movement 2). Each MoFo has a loading prescription, based on the percentage. MoFo alternates on the minute.

Here is a sample program:

FSQ 5-5-5-5-5 @80% of 1RM
PJ 5-5-5-5-5 @80% of 1RM

Load two bars to the appropriate weight, leading with a warm-up to final loading. Set the clock for 10 one-minute intervals. For the starting interval, do 5 FSQ; for the second interval, do 5 PJ; for the third interval, do 5 FSQ; continue to alternate until all the intervals are completed. Anyone who uses this sequence (or others that fall under the same heading), will know why I named it MoFo. This particular programming should only be attempted if one has done the work to develop to this point in the season.

PLEASE NOTE THAT THIS IS THE ACTUAL, UNALTERED PROGRAMMING.
You will see it exactly the way it happened! For example, some days will include "Holiday Special", "Instructor Play" or TBA. The training season between the 2010 and 2011 CrossFit Games was only 50 weeks, so this "year" contains only 50 weeks.

HOW DO YOU PROGRAM FOR THE GAMES?
Programming for CrossFit Games training is intended as preparation for an unknown quantity. Traditional strength and conditioning training is used to develop or support an athlete's capability in another, clearly understood and rule-based sport. For example, a college wrestler may lift and condition for an hour in the morning and in the afternoon, followed by a 3-hour wrestling practice session. The training elements should support overall strength and condition, as demanded by the sport. The requirements are usually straightforward.

BUT HOW DO YOU TRAIN WHEN STRENGTH AND CONDITIONING IS YOUR SPORT?
Step #1: What can the athlete be expected to be able to do?

The CrossFit Games have featured a wide variety of (sometimes unanticipated) requirements. There were long events, like the beach event in 2011 and Camp Pendleton in 2012; skill sets like hand walking; maximum effort lifts under stress; gymnastics skills, adaptive skills and the ability to have very high output.

Step #2: Balanced training.

We tend to think about training in terms of exposure to stimulus and movements. Strength training is the pillar of our system. It takes a very long time to develop strength. Most people make quick progress initially, but slow down as timegoes on. The strength vector in training needs to be consistent and persistent. Applied strength in Olympic weightlifting movements is a time and skill development vector. Consistent drilling of the movement patterns and support movements is essential to development, and creates a foundation required for all other progress. Differentiation between strength (back squat, front squat, deadlift, bench press) and applied strength (snatch, clean, jerk) is needed to cover the variance of demands placed on the athlete by different movements. For example, the athletic requirement for a squat is much lower than for a snatch. The squat is a great support exercise for the snatch, and is foundational to developing the snatch, not the other way around. Gymnastic skills for the CrossFit athlete are developed in a fashion similar to weightlifting. Body weight movements for strength are developed much like the back squat, through loading and repetition.

HOW IS A YEAR OF GAMES TRAINING PROGRAMMING STRUCTURED?

The schedule is created to prepare athletes to be ready to compete in time for the CrossFit Games, which usually take place in mid- to late July of every year. In order to build the base of ability required of a games competitor, the athlete must be able to devote 12 to 20 hours each week to training and training-related items.

Training Focus:

1. Gross Strength.

2. Applied Strength (Olympic Weightlifting).

3. METCON - Intensity Exposure.

- Short: 4 Minutes or less.

- Medium: 4 to 12 minutes.

- Long: 12 to 20 minutes.

- Endurance: 20 to 60 Minutes.

4. Gymnastics.

- Basic Skills.

- Intermediate.

- Applied (used in WOD).

5. Accessory (Farm Boy Power).

For the training season leading up to the 2012 CrossFit Games, the dates were different from the current programming, as follows: Phase I - August 2011 through April 01, 2012; Phase II - April 02, 2012 through May 19, 2012; Phase III - May 20, 2012 through July 01, 2012; Phase IV - July 02, 2012 through July 14, 2012; Phase V (CROSSFIT GAMES 2012) - July 15, 2012 to beginning of 2013 training season.

Our present schedule looks like this:

Phase I: Post-Games August to December is recovery and first part of base building; here we establish a strength cycle that will last until the open. Mid-December to January is a recovery and de-load phase; enjoy the holidays.

Phase II: January to March (beginning of Open).

Phase III: Open to Regionals (depends on year).

Phase IV: Regions to two weeks before the games.

Phase V: Peak and Games.

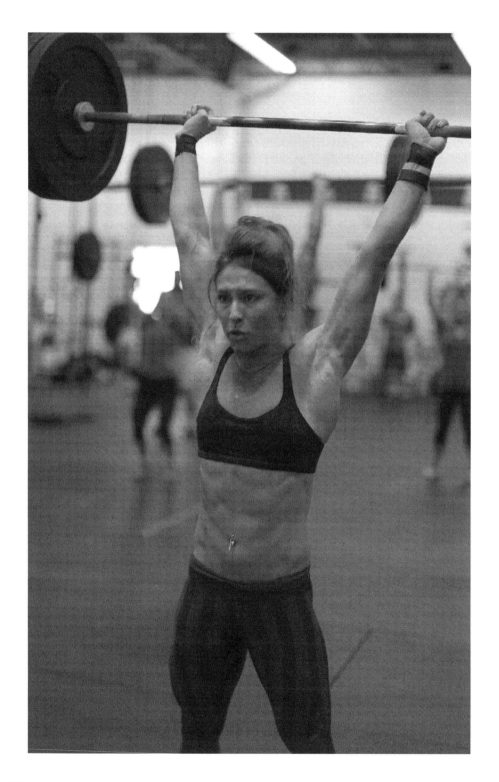

Testimonials

Andrea Ager, CrossFit Athlete & Trainer:

HyperFit programming has changed the way I view training in general. Whether I'm training clients, working out in a biggroup, or following the programming on my own, I know that thinking outside the box is how I remain consistent.

Getting all the lifts done throughout each week, with a steady base of strength-building, gymnastics exercises and short workouts, I feel like I've covered all the domains required. Questioning why, how, or if, gets no results. Practicing all the different skills on a daily basis makes me a more well-rounded athlete.

I've now been able to take the guesswork out of competing. I went from 'hoping I was prepared', to simply knowing I was rehearsed enough for the battle when it mattered.

The volume of strength reps has built a base, and I steadily become more comfortable and consistent, getting to know my body and what I can expect from it during the 'tests of competition.'

Deanna Whiteley, Owner, CrossFit Zone:

I am a box owner, and I was having a hard time being committed to my programming. I found myself being very inconsistent with my training, so I contacted Doug eight months ago. When I started following the HyperFit programming, I found that I was unable to get through the volume, or do the RX weights. I kept plugging through, and rotated between doing RX (where possible) and doing less volume, and then scaling the workouts and doing all the volume.

Within a short few months, I was able to RX most of the weights and do all the volume on the majority of the days. I love following Doug's programming, because it gives me a chance to work on my goals as well as my strengths, with variety.

I don't have to think about what I am doing, I just grab the work for the day and get it done. I feel like this is very important for me, because I can get in my head too much, and better results are achieved when I can stay out of it ;)

I was very surprised at my last competition, that I had gained so much strength from the program. I found the strength

WODs easier than the body weight WODs. For someone my size, it should be opposite.

It is hard to program for CrossFit, because there are so many areas that need to be covered. I feel that Doug has that dialed in. In the 8 months, I have become stronger in every aspect of CrossFit, and maintained momentum in other areas.

Nicole Christensen,
CrossFit Roots/CrossFit HQ Seminar Staff (crossfitroots.com):

I had been doing CrossFit competitively for a few years before I started Doug's program (top 10 at Regionals 2009, 2012). Each year I fell short in the same areas, and while I committed to working on my weaknesses over the following off-season, each year I would come up short the same way, as I tried to create my own piecemeal programming.

Doug's program brought structure and consistency to all areas of a strong GPP program, one that will serve any athlete well, at any competitive level. Having done Doug's system for a year, I had hard numbers to show that what were once weaknesses, had been addressed through consistent and focused practice.

Frank Wray, CrossFit Athlete, Masters Competitor:

I am 49 years old, and a Masters-level competitor. I have been doing CrossFit for a little over a year now, and about 6 months on Doug's system.

I started his programming last August, and went through a shock-and-awe period. I wasn't used to that much volume, and my older body took time to adjust and recover; however, like most of the other athletes, my aerobic and anaerobic capacities have since increased. In addition, all my strength components have improved 25% or more, depending on the movement. I have increased my mobility, as well.

The most important part of my experience has been the mental aspect. Going to Doug's technique camps and watching his approach to each and every movement has been an eye-opener for me. Seeing and applying his philosophy, his approach, and his techniques on coaching, on training, and on life have had a significant impact on my overall fitness, and on all other aspects of my life. I have learned that you can have all the physical tools in the world, but if you can't pair them with the required mental capacity and mental toughness, than your chances of failure increase and your ability to succeed decreases.

Rich Guidotti:

Doug's programming has enabled several people in our gym to see improvements between eight and fifty percent in their level of fitness. We tracked three 2012 CrossFit Open participants. They averaged a 20% performance improvement, leading up to the 2013 CrossFit Open. We not only see this in Open participants, but broadly across all members at our gym.

Doug intelligently applies sound training principles and techniques, and his early adoption of state-of-the-art tools allows his athletes to achieve outstanding results.

In addition to his excellent programming, Doug does a great job analyzing movement faults and explaining corrections in a simple effective manner. I recommend Doug's programming and coaching to anyone looking to increase theiroverall fitness.

Colleen Loughman, mother, wife and CrossFit Athlete:

I thought I kept myself in good shape by jogging, or logging time on elliptical machines. The reality was that my body was very weak. I could barely lift an empty barbell, and my core was so undeveloped that my back was extremely vulnerable to injury.

I knew that this was a special program, an opportunity to be better on many levels. This was about more than just working out. It was about learning and being challenged, both mentally and physically, and achieving goals which, prior to joining HyperFit, I could not have imagined.

Doug's programming, and the professional trainers at HyperFit, are well suited to training elite athletes, and even other trainers. More importantly for me, they also transform ordinary people. HyperFit turned a weak and deteriorating 40-something mom into a strong barbell wrangler who can knock out pull-ups. This kind of trans-formation transcends gym walls. It has made me more capable in all aspects of my life.

Shana Alverson, Owner/Head Trainer, CrossFit East Decatur:

Following HyperFit's (Doug's) programming has been one of the most challenging years of my life. I made a tremendous amount of progress in my snatch, clean and jerk, and finally reached PR in numerous CrossFit benchmarks, even after previously practicing CF for 5 years!

I already had pretty good numbers, but was unsure I could keep up with some of the newer athletes coming to CrossFit, as the sport expanded in recent years. I was able to qualify for the CrossFit Games for the fourth year in a row. Thanks to Doug's programming, not only can I hang with the younger girls, but also continue to grow and thrive as an athlete.

Jen Osborn, CrossFit Athlete:

My goal is to get to the Games! For two years I've tried other coaches, and even coached myself; however, that wasn't enough. I've learned this past year under Doug, that in order for me to reach my goals, I had to really step it up.

Those first couple of months of Doug's programming were eye-opening, for sure! I had a horrible squat, horrible technique on most movements, and most importantly, needed to do much more volume. We are professional athletes - most people think it's insane to train this much.

Today, I'm a completely different athlete and coach. Doug has reason behind all his madness, and I get it! Our bodies are capable of more than you could ever know. Doug's program has pushed me more than anything I previously tried, and I feel very confident going into this season.

Nick Fory, Owner/Operator, Mad City CrossFit; Level 1 Certified Instructor:
Since starting work with HyperFit, I have seen huge gains in every aspect of my training. Raw strength has always been my biggest issue; now my strength numbers are well beyond where I thought they would be at this point. I have always done my own programming in the past, and it is a big relief to not have to worry about it anymore. There are countless WODs that Doug programs, that I would never come close to programming for myself, and I think that's the beauty of HyperFit.

Carla Bezold, CrossFit Athlete:
Since starting HyperFit programming, I've seen substantial increases in my strength and power. More importantly, I have learned to apply that strength and power to a range of tasks and movements, including many I previously had not been exposed to. Every component of the day's training has a purpose, and each day builds on the last. Seeing progress in all areas of my fitness has reminded me why I love to train, to compete, and to test myself every day.

Glissel Soliz, CrossFit Athlete:
It's been an amazing journey since I joined Doug's programming in August, 2012.

I suffered a back injury in January 2012, and lost a lot of strength and confidence in myself, as the injury took me out of training for several months. When I started the programming, I hadn't really lifted since the injury, so my strength numbers were much lower than my maxes.

Fast-forward to the present: my strength has skyrocketed, I'm confident in myself, I am better at BW movements (previously my weakness), I've had no issues with my back and I'm setting PRs on my metcons. I've followed two other programs prior to my injury, and didn't see close to the improvements that I'm seeing now on Doug's system.

Sarah Ralston, CrossFit Athlete:
Doug's programming is absolutely brilliant. Everything is meticulously planned, down to the last skill set, and methodically structured into a framework designed to improve the athlete in every way, to perform well in competition.

It is clear that each aspect of the programming - weights/lifting, WODs and skills - has its own place in the overall long term plan. The WODs/skills are highly varied and never boring. For me as an athlete (not a coach) it's cut and dry: all I have to do is put in the work and reap the results.

CrossFit is evidence-based fitness, and I can speak from personal experience that I have greatly benefitted from this system. I started Doug's programming as a decent athlete (previously in CrossFit for 6 months) but lacking strength, Olympic lifting, and many skills. After another 6 months on his workouts, all my lifts and O-lifts were vastly better, and my benchmark WODs all improved astronomically, as did all my skills. I qualified for Central East Regionals at 36th place, and ended up 21st overall for women (Central East) in 2012, something I didn't think I would ever do. Without a doubt, I owe all this rapid improvement to Doug's programming, and NO WAY would I have been as prepared for competition without it. Going into Regionals, I felt as ready as I could ever be, and I have Doug's programming to thank for it.

Bea Swedlow, CrossFit Athlete:
Testimonials about training are cheap. Results offer the best testimonials.

I walked into HyperFit over five-and-a-half years ago, dreadfully overweight and motivated to transform my life and my level of fitness. Not a day has gone by, that I fail to think about my training, my fitness and my progress.

The numbers don't lie. What I can do today, I could not imagine doing five and a half years ago. The programming and trainers at HyperFit USA, their attention to detail, and their fanaticism about proper form and technique, make this gym something truly special. I make it a habit, when I travel, to visit local CrossFit boxes. I've also participated in a number of certifications. I'm reminded each time how lucky I am, to have one of the best in the business in my backyard.

Josh Pokempner, CrossFit Athlete, Masters Competitor:
On October 5th, 2009, I made a personal declaration that in six months, at my sixtieth birthday, I would be in the best shape ever. I had no idea how I was going to get there, especially since my plan was to follow the same "expert advice" of eat less, exercise more, long slow burning cardio treadmill exercise, weight machines and low fat nutritional diet, all which consistently failed in the past.

What was different this time, was Doug Chapman. On that same day in 2009, I walked into Doug's gym solely because of its convenient location to my office, with no clue about him, his gym, process or philosophy. He told me I only needed to do two things to reach my goal: "Show up and do as you're told". Fair enough, I showed up and did as I was told. Six months later, I was a different man: 30 pounds lighter, 10% body fat, rock-star lipids, deadlift twice my body weight. All this was accomplished with less (but more efficient) exercise, and eating smart without deprivation. An unexpected, but welcome, bonus is the overall improvement - feeling great and participating more in life. This wasn't just about selfesteem, but more about truly feeling vibrant and fit for life's challenges.

Eric Haskins, Team Captain, Boise State Men's Ice Hockey Club:
Reflecting on Douglas Chapman (or "The Wizard of Wodz", as my brother and I call him), and his prescription for gains and pains, I must say that, as much as I hate it, I really love it!

Since I started training with Doug Chapman and his stable of talented and mentally capable freak-shows, I have been challenged mentally and physically in ways I have never experienced before.

In my previous life, before all of this madness, I was a professional snowboard racer for six years, and was named to the US Project Gold Snowboard Team at age 18. I trained with members of the US Snowboard team the first part of my career, then took the opportunity to move to Calgary, AB, to train with the Canadian National Development Team at theCanadian Olympic Training Center. During this period, I competed on the world snowboard tour circuit, and worked with North America's elite strength coaches in state-of-the-art facilities. In 2009, after qualifying for the snowboard World Cup tour, I lost my spot due to poor performance in the Europa Cup competition in Europe. I had a lingering stress fracture in my leg prior to the event, and separated my shoulder during my first round in Switzerland. Upon my return home, the doctors told me that I had accumulated too many injuries, and qualifying for the 2010 Olympics was almost impossible. After four shoulder operations, my body had enough, and I would never compete again. I was directed to prepare for my final surgery: two full shoulder replacements by the age of 30.

I ignored this surgical advice, retired from snowboarding, and went back to ice hockey, a sport I played in my youth (and took up again in Canada). I was subsequently recruited by Boise State University. I have been Captain of the Boise State hockey team for 3 years now, and every day has been a fight against the doctors' verdict. HyperFit programming has been the opposite of all the other training in my previous athletic career. It is the most difficult program I have ever experienced. The physical challenges have tested my mental capacity in ways I'd never faced before. I often ask myself, "How the hell did he come up with this? How is it going to benefit me, and why am I going to do this?!"

It is only when we are late in a game, down 3-2, shorthanded on the penalty kill, that I realize why this system is so effective. I can picture Doug's mad-scientist smile in some dark and evil corner, as he programs for next week. It is then that I have enough in the tank, and believe that just maybe, I can make one last push down the ice with the puck, instead of dumping it. I know now that pain is only temporary, and I make the choice to push through, regardless of circumstances, to turn things around for my team.

Most importantly, Doug's HyperFit programming has taught me to believe in myself and dictate my own destiny. Modern sports medicine condemned me to a sedentary life, after a good run in my early twenties. With the support of the HyperFit community and the coaching from Douglas (the WoW), Michael O'Brian (M.O.B), and Jeff (Negative Nancy), I can live on my own terms. I'm stronger mentally and physically now than I've ever been, thanks to the effectiveness of HyperFit training.

There are some who say that I'm crazy to do all this, but I just laugh. Such people sit on the sidelines, never discovering their full potential. To them, it may look like a barbell that's "too heavy", but it may be any aspect of their life. I can either grab it with my ripped and bleeding hands (which most definitely will hurt like hell), or I can throw in the towel and call it a day, hiding behind petty excuses. Doug would simply say: "Do it, and Do it Now!"

Acknowledgement

It is hard to list everyone who deserves a place here. There are too many, but room only for a few.

First and foremost would be my father. He taught me to think independently, and to question conventional wisdom. This practice yielded great returns, and is essential to living free.

Greg Glassman created the foundation upon which I have built my training system. He shaped my ideas about what was possible. He created an organization where what works is adopted, and what fails is discarded. He created a meritocracy in the fitness industry; a body of practice that focuses on results, and not on the latest gadget or infomercial.

My clients push me to experiment and improvise; they are a major source of inspiration. They have used some good (and not so good) programming over the years. Without them, my own learning curve from 2003 would have been much slower and more difficult.

A note of profound gratitude goes to the 2011 Games Central East Regional Championship team: Johnny Kozlowski, Anna Rode, Matt Young, Merrill Mullis, Dani Urcuyo and Julie Foucher. They rekindled my faith in the human work ethic, and the individual drive to succeed.

Special thanks go out to my staff, for looking after the shop and supporting our athletes.

Finally, I want to thank Hunter, my son. He taught me more in six years than I thought possible. He inspires me to be a better person.

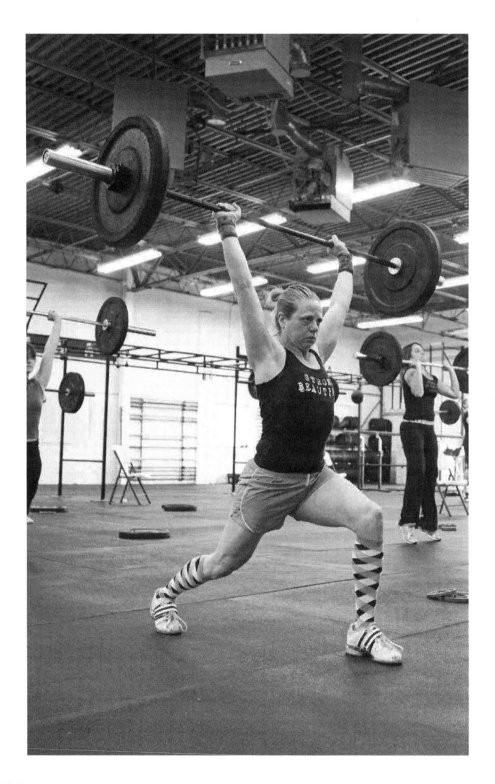

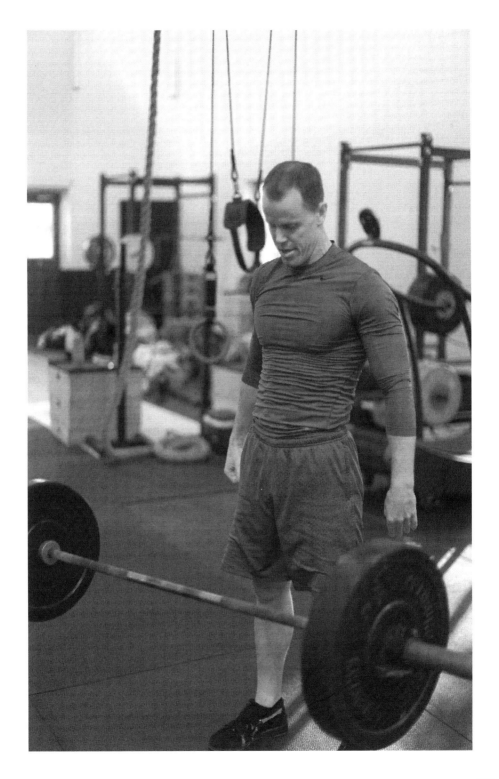

Week 1

	SUNDAY 7/31	MONDAY 8/1	TUESDAY 8/2
WARM UP	Run: 400 **Then 4 Rounds of** :15 Jumping Jack :15 Squat :15 Mountain Climber :15 Jump Squat	*Instructor Lead* **3 Rounds of** Lunge: 20ft Inch Worm: 20ft Hand Release Push Up: 15 AbMat: 15	*Instructor Lead* 30/20/30 **Then 5 Rounds of** Hand Release Push Up: 15 AbMat: 15 Split Squat: 20
EQUIPMENT	Sled: 35/25 BB: #135/#95 Dynamax #20/#14	KB 24/16 Slammer 30/15	Low Box DB #35/#25
WOD	**A1:** Sled 100 (Pace) **A2:** Wall Ball (Score) **A3:** Deadlift (Score) *AMRAP: 13 Minutes*	Run: 200 Swing: 15 Slam: 15 *5 Rounds for time -* *10:00 Time Cap*	Low Box Jump: 50 Pull Up: 40 FSQ: 30 Burpee: 20 Thruster: 10 *For time*
LIFTING/ SKILL DEV	Instructor lead roll/stretch	Instructor lead roll/stretch	Instructor lead roll/stretch
GAMES Phase I	Recovery - Training Optional	Recovery - Training Optional	Recovery - Training Optional

NOTES

WEDNESDAY 8/3	THURSDAY 8/4	FRIDAY 8/5	SATURDAY 8/6
Row: 1000 30/20/30 **Then** Run: 50 (technique) Walk: 50 *AMRAP: 10 Minutes* Pro Agility 5 Min Right 5 Min Left	Run: 400 *Then Instructor Lead* 30/20/30 **Then** *Cindy*	*Instructor Lead* 30/20/30 HRPU: 20 AbMat: 20 Split Squat: 20	Run: 400 30/20/30
BB: #185/#135	BB #135/#95 AbMat	BB: #135/#95	BB 95/65
Power Clean Burpee *21, 15, 9 for time*	DL: 25 AbMAt: 25 *5 Rounds for time*	*7 Rounds of* Pull Up: 7 OHS: 7	*Thunder* Pull Up: 5 Push Press: 10 Thruster: 15 *AMRAP: 20 Minutes*
Instructor lead roll/stretch	Instructor lead roll/stretch	Instructor lead roll/stretch	Instructor lead roll/stretch
Recovery - Training Optional	**Recovery - Training Optional**	**Recovery - Training Optional**	**Recovery - Training Optional**

NOTES

23

WEEK 1 -
SUN JUL 31 2011

PHASE I:
Recovery - Training Optional

WARMUP:
Run: 400
Then 4 Rounds of
:15 Jumping Jack
:15 Squat
:15 Mountain Climber
:15 Jump Squat

EQUIPMENT:
Sled: 35/25;
Dynamax #20/#14;
BB: #135/#95

WOD:
P1: Sled 100 (Pace)
P2: Wall Ball (Score)
P3: Deadlift (Score)
AMRAP: 13 Minutes

LIFTING/SKILL DEV:
Instructor lead roll/stretch

WEEK 1 -
MON AUG 01 2011

PHASE I:
Recovery - Training Optional

WARMUP:
Instructor Lead
3 Rounds of
Lunge: 20ft
Inch Worm: 20ft
Hand Release Push Up: 15
AbMat: 15

EQUIPMENT:
KB 24/16; Slammer 30/15

WOD:
Run: 200
Russian Swing: 15
Slam: 15
5 Rounds for time -
10 Minute Time Cap

LIFTING/SKILL DEV:
Instructor lead roll/stretch

WEEK 1 -
TUE AUG 02 2011

PHASE I:
Recovery - Training Optional

WARMUP:
Instructor Lead
30/20/30 -
30 Air Squats/20 Roll Outs/
30 Overhead Squats w/PVC
Then 5 Rounds of
Hand Release Push Up: 10
AbMat: 15
Split Squat: 20

EQUIPMENT:
6in Low Box;
Dumbbells #35/#25

WOD:
Low Box Jump: 50
Pull Up: 40
FSQ: 30
Burpee: 20
Thruster: 10
For time

LIFTING/SKILL DEV:
Instructor lead roll/stretch

WEEK 1 -
WED AUG 03 2011

PHASE I:
Recovery - Training Optional

WARMUP:
Row: 1000
30/20/30
Then
Run: 50
(technique - P.O.S.E. Drill)
Walk: 50
AMRAP: 10 Minutes
Then
Pro Agility
5 Min Right
5 Min Left

EQUIPMENT:
BB #185/#135

WOD:
Power Clean
Burpee
21, 15, 9 for time

LIFTING/SKILL DEV:
Instructor lead roll/stretch

WEEK 1 -
THU AUG 04 2011

PHASE I:
Recovery - Training Optional

WARMUP:
Run: 400
Then Instructor Lead
30/20/30
Then 5 Rounds of
Cindy

EQUIPMENT:
BB #135/#95; AbMat

WOD:
DL: 25
AbMat: 25
5 Rounds for time

LIFTING/SKILL DEV:
Instructor lead roll/stretch

WEEK 1 -
FRI AUG 05 2011

PHASE I:
Recovery - Training Optional

WARMUP:
Instructor Lead
30/20/30
HRPU: 20
AbMat: 20
Split Squat: 20

EQUIPMENT:
BB #135/#95

WOD:
7 Rounds of
Pull Up: 7
OHS: 7

LIFTING/SKILL DEV:
Instructor lead roll/stretch

WEEK 1 -
SAT AUG 06 2011

PHASE I:
Recovery - Training Optional

WARMUP:
Run: 400
30/20/30

EQUIPMENT:
BB #95/#65

WOD:
Thunder:
Pull Up: 5
Push Press: 10
Thruster: 15
AMRAP: 20 Minutes

LIFTING/SKILL DEV:
Instructor lead roll/stretch

NOTES

27

Week 2

	SUNDAY 8/7	MONDAY 8/8	TUESDAY 8/9
WARM UP	*Instructor Lead* **4 Rounds of** :15 Jumping Jack :15 Squat :15 Mountain Climber :15 Jump Squat **Then** 30/20/30	**Instructor Lead** Run: 400 30/20/30 Clean and Jerk Skills (empty BB)	*Instructor Lead* 30/20/30 *Then 4 Rounds of* Sit Up: 10 Push Up (HR): 20
EQUIPMENT	Butcher: 90/70 BB: 65/45 BB: 135/95	BB: #155/#105	BB: #135/#95
W O D	**A1** : Butcher HiPush: 50 **A2** : PP (Score) **A3** : PCL (Score) *AMRAP: 15 Minutes*	CL: 1 FSQ: 2 Jerk: 1 *AMRAP: 20 Minutes*	Run: 100 Squats: 20 *5 Rounds for time*
LIFTING/ SKILL DEV	Instructor lead roll/stretch	Instructor lead roll/stretch	Instructor lead roll/stretch
GAMES Phase I	Recovery - Training Optional	All	All
Power Hour All lifts @80% of 1RM		BSQ 5 x 5 Press 5 x 5 **Then** Sled Drag: 800 (#135/ #90) *for time*	FSQ 5 x 5 Push Jerk 5 x 5 **Then** Butcher HiPush: 25 (135/90) Run: 50 *AMRAP: 10 Minutes*

WEDNESDAY 8/10	THURSDAY 8/11	FRIDAY 8/12	SATURDAY 8/13
Run: 400 30/20/30 **Then** Run: 50 Lunge: 50 *AMRAP: 10* *Minutes*	*Instructor Lead* Row: 1000 30/20/30 **Then 4 Rounds of** Jumping Jack: 30 (4ct) Push Up (HR): 10	Run: 400 **Then Instructor Lead** *4 Rounds of* 8-Count Body Builder: 10 AbMat: 20	**4 Rounds of** :15 Jumping Jack :15 Squat :15 Mountain Climber :15 Jump Squat
Box: 20in Rings	Dynamax Ball: 20/14		BB: 255/185 BB: 115/75 Box: 24/20 DB: 45/35
Ring Row: 12 Ring Push Up: 12	Wall Ball: 15 Burpee: 15 *5 Rounds for time*	Lunge: 25yds Run: 50yds *AMRAP: 10 Minutes -* *Rest 5:00* *Then* Pull Up: 5 Push Up: 10 *AMRAP: 10 Minutes*	Deadlifts: 20 Run 400m KB swings: 20 Run 400m Overhead Squats: 20 Run 400m Burpees: 20 Run 400m Pullups (C2B): 20 Run 400m Box jumps: 20 Run 400m DB Squat Cleans: 20 Run 400m
Instructor lead roll/stretch	Instructor lead roll/stretch	Instructor lead roll/stretch	Instructor lead roll/stretch
All	**All**	**Class Only**	**Rest**
DL 5 x 5 Split Jerk 5 x 5 **Then** Sled Drag: 800 (#135/#90) for time	OHS 5 x 5 Pull Up 5 x 5 (Strict) **Then** Butcher HiPush: 25 (135/90) Run 50 *AMRAP: 10 Minutes*		

WEEK 2 - SUN AUG 07 2011

PHASE I:
Recovery - Training Optional

WARMUP:
Instructor Lead
4 Rounds of
:15 Jumping Jack
:15 SQT
:15 MC
:15 JSQT
Then
30/20/30

EQUIPMENT:
Butcher: 90/70; BB: 65/45;
BB: 135/95

WOD:
P1: Butcher Hi Push: 50
P2: PP (Score)
P3: PCL (Score)
AMRAP: 15 Minutes

LIFTING/SKILL DEV:
Instructor lead roll/stretch

WEEK 2 - MON AUG 08 2011

PHASE I:
Games Track Athletes - All

WARMUP:
Instructor Lead
Run: 400
30/20/30
Clean and Jerk Skills
w/Empty Barbell

EQUIPMENT:
BB: #155/#105

WOD:
CL: 1
FSQ: 2
Jerk: 1
AMRAP: 20 Minutes

LIFTING/SKILL DEV:
Instructor lead roll/stretch
GAMES: After Class

POWER HOUR:
BSQ 5 x 5 @80% of 1RM
Press 5 x 5 @80% of 1RM
Then
Sled Drag: 800 -
#135/#90 added to Sled
For time

WEEK 2 -
TUE AUG 09 2011

PHASE I:
Games Track Athletes - All

WARMUP:
Instructor Lead
30/20/30
Then 4 Rounds of
Sit Up: 10
Push Up (HR): 20

EQUIPMENT:
BB #135/#95

WOD:
Run: 100
Squats: 20
5 Rounds for time

LIFTING/SKILL DEV:
Instructor lead roll/stretch

GAMES:
After Class

POWER HOUR:
FSQ 5 x 5 @80% of 1RM
Push Jerk 5 x 5
@80% of 1RM
Then
Butcher Hi Push: 25yds
(#135/#90)
Run 50
AMRAP: 10 Minutes

WEEK 2 -
WED AUG 10 2011

PHASE I:
Games Track Athletes - All

WARMUP:
Run: 400
30/20/30
Then
Run: 50
Lunge: 50
AMRAP: 10 Minutes

EQUIPMENT:
Box: 20in; Rings

WOD:
Ring Row: 12
Ring Push Up: 12

LIFTING/SKILL DEV:
Instructor lead roll/stretch

GAMES:
After Class

POWER HOUR:
DL 5 x 5 @80% of 1RM
Split Jerk 5 x 5 @80% of 1RM

Sled Drag: 800 - #135/#90
For time

31

WEEK 2 -
THU AUG 11 2011

PHASE I:
Games Track Athletes - All

WARMUP:
Instructor Lead
Row: 1000
30/20/30
Then 5 Rounds of
Jumping Jack: 30 (4-count)
Push Up (HR): 10

EQUIPMENT:
Dynamax Ball: #20/#14

WOD:
Wall Ball: 15
Burpee: 15
5 Rounds for time

LIFTING/SKILL DEV:
Instructor lead roll/stretch

GAMES:
After Class

POWER HOUR:
OHS 5 x 5 @80% of 1RM
Pull Up 5 x 5 (Strict - No Kip)
Then
Butcher Hi Push: 25 (135/90)
Run 50
AMRAP: 10 Minutes

WEEK 2 -
FRI AUG 12 2011

PHASE I:
Games Track Athletes -
Class Only

WARMUP:
Run: 400
Then Instructor Lead
3 Rounds of
8 Count Body Builder: 10
AbMat: 20

WOD:
Lunge: 25yds
Run: 50yds
AMRAP: 10 Minutes
Rest 5:00
Then
Pull Up: 5
Push Up: 10
AMRAP: 10 Minutes

LIFTING/SKILL DEV:
Instructor lead roll/stretch

GAMES:
Class Only

WEEK 2 -
SAT AUG 13 2011

PHASE I:
Games Track Athletes -
Rest Day

WARMUP:
4 Rounds of
:15 Jumping Jack
:15 SQT
:15 MC
:15 JSQT

EQUIPMENT:
BB: 255/185; BB 115/75;
Box: 24/20; DB 45/35

WOD:
Deadlifts: 20
Run 400m
KB swings: 20
Run 400m
Overhead Squats: 20
Run 400m
Burpees: 20
Run 400m
Pullups (C2B): 20
Run 400m
Box jumps: 20
Run 400m
DB Squat Cleans: 20
Run 400m
For time

LIFTING/SKILL DEV:
Instructor lead roll/stretch

Week 3

	SUNDAY 8/14	MONDAY 8/15	TUESDAY 8/16
WARM UP	*Instructor Lead* 30/20/30 **Then 5 Rounds of** HRPU: 10 AbMat: 20	Run: 400 **Then** *Instructor Lead* 30/20/30 **Then 3 Rounds of** HRPU: 10 T2B: 10 Dip: 10	*Instructor Lead* 30/20/30 **Then 5 Rounds of** HRPU: 10 AbMat: 20
EQUIPMENT	Slammer #50/#30 Sandbag: 70/50 Blue 6in Box	BB: 95/65	KB 28kg/16kg
W O D	**A1**: Run 100 **A2**: Sandbag Thruster (Score) **A3**: Low Box Jump (Score) *AMRAP: 12 Minutes*	Run: 400 PSN: 15 *5 Rounds for time*	American Swing: 21 Burpee: 15 Pull Up: 9 *3 Rounds for time*
LIFTING/ SKILL DEV	Instructor lead roll/stretch	Instructor lead roll/stretch	Instructor lead roll/stretch
GAMES Phase I	All	All	All
Power Hour All lifts @80% of 1RM		FSQ 3-3-3-3-3 Push Jerk 3-3-3-3-3 **Then** Butcher HiPush: 25 (135/90) Run 50 *AMRAP: 10 Minutes*	DL 3-3-3-3-3 Split Jerk 3-3-3-3-3 **Then** Sled Drag: 800 (#135/#90) *for time*

WEDNESDAY 8/17	THURSDAY 8/18	FRIDAY 8/19	SATURDAY 8/20
Run: 400 **Then Instructor Lead** 30/20/30 **Then 3 Rounds of** HRPU: 10 T2B: 10 Dip: 10	*Instructor Lead* 30/20/30 **Then 5 Rounds of** HRPU: 10 AbMat: 20	Run: 400 *Then Instructor Lead* 30/20/30 *Then 3 Rounds of* HRPU: 10 T2B: 10 Dip: 10	*Instructor Lead* 30/20/30 **Then 5 Rounds of** HRPU: 10 AbMat: 20
Slammer #30/20	BB: 115/75	BB 155/105	BB 135/95
Run: 800 **Then** Ball Slam Wall Ball *21, 15, 9 for time*	Run: 400 Thruster: 15 Push Jerk: 10 Ring Dip: 5 *5 Rounds for time*	Run: 400 Clean and Jerk: 12 *7 Rounds for time*	*Isabel* *Snatch version*
Instructor lead roll/stretch	Instructor lead roll/stretch	Instructor lead roll/stretch	Instructor lead roll/stretch
All	**All**	**Rest**	**All**
OHS 3-3-3-3-3 Pull Up 3-3-3-3-3 (Strict) **Then** Butcher HiPush: 25 (135/90) Run 50 *AMRAP: 10 Minutes*	BSQ 3-3-3-3-3 Press 3-3-3-3-3 *Then* Sled Drag: 800 (#135/#90) *time*		

NOTES

_____

_____

_____

_____

_____

35

WEEK 3 -
SUN AUG 14 2011

PHASE I:
Games Track Athletes - All

WARMUP:
Instructor Lead
30/20/30
Then 5 Rounds of
HRPU: 10
AbMat: 20

EQUIPMENT:
Slammer #50/#30;
Sandbag: 70/50; Blue 6in Box

WOD:
P1: Run 100 w/Ball
P2: Sandbag Thruster (Score)
P3: Low Box Jump (Score)
AMRAP: 12 Minutes

LIFTING/SKILL DEV:
Instructor lead roll/stretch

WEEK 3 -
TUE AUG 16 2011

PHASE I:
Games Track Athletes - All

WARMUP:
Instructor Lead
30/20/30
Then 5 Rounds of
HRPU: 10
AbMat: 20

EQUIPMENT:
KB 28kg/16kg

WOD:
American Swing: 21
Burpee: 15
Pull Up: 9
3 Rounds for time

LIFTING/SKILL DEV:
Instructor lead roll/stretch

GAMES:
After Class

POWER HOUR:
DL 3-3-3-3-3 @90% of 1RM
Split Jerk 3-3-3-3-3
@90% of 1RM
Then
Sled Drag: 800 - #135/#90
For time

WEEK 3 -
TUE AUG 16 2011

PHASE I:
Games Track Athletes - All

WARMUP:
Instructor Lead
30/20/30
Then 5 Rounds of
HRPU: 10
AbMat: 20

EQUIPMENT:
KB 28kg/16kg

WOD:
American Swing: 21
Burpee: 15
Pull Up: 9
3 Rounds for time

LIFTING/SKILL DEV:
Instructor lead roll/stretch

GAMES:
After Class

POWER HOUR:
DL 3-3-3-3-3 @90% of 1RM
Split Jerk 3-3-3-3-3
@90% of 1RM
Then
Sled Drag: 800 - #135/#90
For time

WEEK 3 -
WED AUG 17 2011

PHASE I:
Games Track Athletes - All

WARMUP:
Run: 400
Then Instructor Lead
30/20/30
Then 3 Rounds of
HRPU: 10
T2B: 10
Dip: 10

EQUIPMENT:
Slammer #30/20
WOD:
Run: 800
Then
Ball Slam
Wall Ball
21, 15, 9 for time

LIFTING/SKILL DEV:
Instructor lead roll/stretch

GAMES:
After Class

POWER HOUR:
OHS 3-3-3-3-3 @90% of 1RM
Pull Up 3-3-3-3-3 (Strict)
Then
Butcher Hi Push: 25 (135/90)
Run 50
AMRAP: 10 Minutes

**WEEK 3 -
THU AUG 18 2011**

PHASE I:
Games Track Athletes - All

WARMUP:
Instructor Lead
30/20/30
Then 5 Rounds of
HRPU: 10
AbMat: 20

EQUIPMENT:
BB: #115/75

WOD:
Run: 400
Thruster: 15
Push Jerk: 10
Ring Dip: 5
5 Rounds for time

LIFTING/SKILL DEV:
Instructor lead roll/stretch

GAMES:
After Class

POWER HOUR:
BSQ 3-3-3-3-3 @90% of 1RM
Press 3-3-3-3-3 @90% of 1RM
Then
Sled Drag: 800 - #135/#90
For time

**WEEK 3 -
FRI AUG 19 2011**

PHASE I:
Games Track Athletes -
Rest Day

WARMUP:
Run: 400
Then Instructor Lead
30/20/30
Then 3 Rounds of
HRPU: 10
T2B: 10
Dip: 10

EQUIPMENT:
BB: 155/105

WOD:
Run: 400
Clean and Jerk: 12
7 Rounds for time

LIFTING/SKILL DEV:
Instructor lead roll/stretch

GAMES:
Class Only

WEEK 3 -
SAT AUG 20 2011

PHASE I:
Games Track Athletes - All

WARMUP:
Instructor Lead
30/20/30
Then 5 Rounds of
HRPU: 10
AbMat: 20

EQUIPMENT: BB: 135/95

WOD:
Isabel - Squat Snatch version

LIFTING/SKILL DEV:
Instructor lead roll/stretch

Week 4

	SUNDAY 8/21	MONDAY 8/22	TUESDAY 8/23
WARM UP	*Instructor Lead* 30/20/30 **Then 4 Rounds of** Jumping Jack (4ct): 10 HR Push Up: 10 AbMat: 10	*Instructor Lead* 30/20/30 **Then 3 Rounds of** *Cindy*	*Instructor Lead* 30/20/30 **Then 4 Rounds of** Jumping Jack (4ct): 10 HR Push Up: 10 AbMat: 10
EQUIPMENT	Slammer: #30/#20 Dynamax: #20/#14	You	BB #135/#95
WOD	**A1** : Run: 200 **A2** : Ball Slam (Score) **A3** : Wall Ball (Score) *AMRAP: 12 Minutes*	Run: 100 Jog: 100 *AMRAP: 10 Minutes - Rest 3:00* **Then** Pull Up: 5 Push Up: 10 Squat: 15 *AMRAP: 10 Minutes*	Clean: 7 Push Jerk: 7 *AMRAP: 3 Minutes - Rest 1:00 - 5 Rounds*
LIFTING/ SKILL DEV	Instructor lead roll/stretch	Instructor lead roll/stretch	Instructor lead roll/stretch
GAMES Phase I	Rest	All	All
Power Hour All lifts Establish 1-Rep Max		DL 1-1-1-1-1-1-1 Split Jerk 1-1-1-1-1-1-1 **Then** Sled Drag: 800 (#135/#90) *for time*	OHS 1-1-1-1-1-1-1 Pull Up 1-1-1-1-1-1-1 (Strict) **Then** Butcher HiPush: 25 (135/90) Run 50 *AMRAP: 10 Minutes*

NOTES

WEDNESDAY 8/24	THURSDAY 8/25	FRIDAY 8/26	SATURDAY 8/27
Instructor Lead 30/20/30 *Then 3 Rounds of* **Cindy**	*Instructor Lead* 30/20/30 **Then 4 Rounds of** Jumping Jack (4ct): 10 HR Push Up: 10 AbMat: 10	*Instructor Lead* 30/20/30 **Then 3 Rounds of** **Cindy**	*Instructor Lead* 30/20/30 **Then 4 Rounds of** Jumping Jack (4ct): 10 HR Push Up: 10 AbMat: 10
KB: 24kg/16kg Slammer: #30/#20 DB: #35/#25	Dynamax #20/#14	BB: #95/#65 Slammer: #30/#20	BB: #225/#155 Box 24in/20in
Swing: 30 Slam: 20 Thruster: 10 *AMRAP: 30 Minutes*	Wall Ball: 15 Burpee: 15 *5 Rounds for time*	PSN: 10 Slam: 12 *5 Rounds for time*	*Roy* Deadlift: 15 Box Jump: 20 Pull Up: 25 *5 Rounds for time*
Instructor lead roll/stretch	Instructor lead roll/stretch	Instructor lead roll/stretch	Instructor lead roll/stretch
All	**All**	**Rest**	**All**
BSQ 1-1-1-1-1-1-1 Press 1-1-1-1-1-1-1 **Then** Sled Drag: 800 (#135/#90) *for time*	FSQ 1-1-1-1-1-1-1 Push Jerk 1-1-1-1-1-1-1 **Then** Butcher HiPush: 25 (135/90) Run 50 *AMRAP: 10 Minutes*		

NOTES

_____

_____

_____

WEEK 4 -
SUN AUG 21 2011

PHASE I:
Games Track Athletes -
Rest Day

WARMUP:
Instructor Lead
30/20/30
Then 4 Rounds of
Jumping Jack (4ct): 10
HR Push Up: 10
AbMat: 10

EQUIPMENT:
Slammer: #30/#20;
Dynamax: #20/#14

WOD:
P1: Run: 200
P2: Ball Slam (Score)
P3: Wall Ball (Score)
AMRAP: 12 Minutes

LIFTING/SKILL DEV:
Instructor lead roll/stretch

WEEK 4 -
MON AUG 22 2011

PHASE I:
Games Track Athletes - All

WARMUP:
Instructor Lead
30/20/30
Then 3 Rounds of
Cindy

EQUIPMENT: You

WOD:
Run: 100yds
Jog: 100yds
AMRAP: 10 Minutes
Rest 3:00
Then
Pull Up: 5
Push Up: 10
Squat: 15
AMRAP: 10 Minutes

LIFTING/SKILL DEV:
Instructor lead roll/stretch

POWER HOUR:
DL 1-1-1-1-1-1-1
Establish 1 Rep Max
Split Jerk 1-1-1-1-1-1-1
Establish 1 Rep Max
Then
Sled Drag: 800 - #135/#90
For time

WEEK 4 - TUES AUG 23 2011

PHASE I:
Games Track Athletes - All

WARMUP:
Instructor Lead
30/20/30
Then 4 Rounds of
Jumping Jack (4ct): 10
HR Push Up: 10
AbMat: 10

EQUIPMENT:
BB #135/#95

WOD:
Clean: 7
Push Jerk: 7
AMRAP: 3 Minutes -
Rest 1:00 - 5 Rounds

LIFTING/SKILL DEV:
Instructor lead roll/stretch

POWER HOUR:
OHS 1-1-1-1-1-1-1
Establish 1 Rep Max
Pull Up 1-1-1-1-1-1-1
(Strict)
Then
Butcher Hi Push: 25yds
(135/90)
Run 50
AMRAP: 10 Minutes

WEEK 4 - WED AUG 24 2011

PHASE I:
Games Track Athletes - All

WARMUP:
Instructor Lead
30/20/30
Then 3 Rounds of
Cindy

EQUIPMENT:
KB: 24kg/16kg;
Slammer: #30/#20;
DB: #35/#25

WOD:
Russian Swing: 30
Slam: 20
Thruster: 10
AMRAP: 30 Minutes

LIFTING/SKILL DEV:
Instructor lead roll/stretch

POWER HOUR:
BSQ 1-1-1-1-1-1-1
Establish 1 Rep Max
Press 1-1-1-1-1-1-1
Establish 1 Rep Max
Then
Sled Drag: 800 - #135/#90
For time

WEEK 4 -
THU AUG 25 2011

PHASE I:
Games Track Athletes - All

WARMUP:
Instructor Lead
30/20/30
Then 4 Rounds of
Jumping Jack (4ct): 10
HR Push Up: 10
AbMat: 10

EQUIPMENT:
Dynamax #20/#14

WOD:
Wall Ball: 15
Burpee: 15
5 Rounds for time

LIFTING/SKILL DEV:
Instructor lead roll/stretch

POWER HOUR:
FSQ 1-1-1-1-1-1-1
Establish 1 Rep Max
Push Jerk 1-1-1-1-1-1-1
Establish 1 Rep Max
Then
Butcher Hi Push: 25yds
(135/90)
Run: 50yds
AMRAP: 10 Minutes

WEEK 4 -
FRI AUG 26 2011

PHASE I:
Games Track Athletes -
Rest Day

WARMUP:
Instructor Lead
30/20/30
Then 3 Rounds of
Cindy

EQUIPMENT:
BB: #95/#65;
Slammer: #30/#20

WOD:
PSN: 10
Slam: 12
5 Rounds for time

LIFTING/SKILL DEV:
Instructor lead roll/stretch

WEEK 4 -
SAT AUG 27 2011

PHASE I:
Games Track Athletes - All

WARMUP:
Instructor Lead
30/20/30
Then 4 Rounds of
Jumping Jack (4ct): 10
HR Push Up: 10
AbMat: 10

EQUIPMENT:
BB: #225/#155; Box 24in/20in

WOD:
Roy:
Deadlift: 15
Box Jump: 20
Pull Up: 25
5 Rounds for time

LIFTING/SKILL DEV:
Instructor lead roll/stretch

Week 5

	SUNDAY 8/28	MONDAY 8/29	TUESDAY 8/30
WARM UP	30/20/30 **Then 4 Rounds of** :15 Jumping Jack :15 Squat :15 Mountain Climber :15 Jump Squat	*Instructor Lead* 30/20/30 **Then w/Bar** *Barbell Skills Complex* **5 Rounds of** DL: 3 CL: 3 FSQ: 3 PJ: 3 OHS: 3 PSN: 3	*Instructor Lead* 30/20/30 **Then 3 Rounds of** *Cindy*
EQUIPMENT	Butcher #50/#30 Box 24/20	BB 225/#155 BB #135/#95	KB: 24kg/16kg Dynamax #20/#14
WOD	**A1** : Butcher HiPush: 50yds **A2** : Box Jump (Score) **A3** : Push Press (Score) *AMRAP: 20 Minutes*	DL: 12 PJ: 10 *5 Rounds for time*	Swing: 50 Wall Ball: 20 *5 Rounds for time*
LIFTING/ SKILL DEV	Instructor lead roll/stretch	Instructor lead roll/stretch	Instructor lead roll/stretch
GAMES Phase I	Rest	All	All
Power Hour		Zercher Squat: 5-5-5-5-5 HSPU 5-5-5-5-5 (Strict) Sprint: 100yds - *Rest 1:00* *- 10 Rounds*	Sled Pull: 100 (#135/#90) Sled Pull Backwards: 100 *AMRAP: 10 Minutes* **Then** Farmer's Walk: 100yds - (2) 32kg KB Run: 200 *AMRAP: 10 Minutes*

WEDNESDAY 8/31	THURSDAY 9/1	FRIDAY 9/2	SATURDAY 9/3
Instructor Lead	*Instructor Lead*	*Instructor Lead*	Run: 400
30/20/30	30/20/30	30/20/30	30/20/30
Then w/Bar	**Then 3 Rounds of**	**Then w/bar**	
Barbell Skills Complex	*Cindy*	*Barbell Skills Complex*	
5 Rounds of		**3 Rounds of**	
DL: 3		OHS: 3	
CL: 3		PSNBAL: 3	
FSQ: 3		HSNBAL: 3	
PP: 3		SNBAL: 3	
OHS: 3		*Then 3 Rounds of*	
PSN: 3		HSN: P1: 3	
		HSN: P2: 3	
		HSN: P3: 3	
BB: #95/#65	BB: #225/#155	BB + Weights	BB #95/#65
Box: 24/20			
Push Press: 7	***Tabata** - :20/:10 x 16*	SN: 1 *EMOTM for 20 Minutes*	***Murph***
Box Jump: 7	DL		
Pull-Up: 7	Burpee		
AMRAP: 15 Minutes	*Alternate between*		
	exercises - Score each		
Instructor lead roll/stretch	Instructor lead roll/stretch	Instructor lead roll/stretch	Instructor lead roll/stretch

All	All	Rest	All
Lunge 25yds (95/65)	FSQ: Max (#135/#95)		
Run: 50yds	Run: 200		
AMRAP: 20 Minutes	*AMRAP: 15 Minutes*		

WEEK 5 -
SUN AUG 28 2011

PHASE I:
Games Track Athletes -
Rest Day

WARMUP:
30/20/30
Then 4 Rounds of
:15 Jumping Jack
:15 Squat
:15 Mountain Climber
:15 Jump Squat

EQUIPMENT:
Butcher #50/#30; Box 24/20

WOD:
P1: Push Butcher: 50yds
P2: Box Jump (Score)
P3: Push Press (Score)
AMRAP: 20 Minutes

LIFTING/SKILL DEV:
Instructor lead roll/stretch

WEEK 5 -
MON AUG 29 2011

PHASE I:
Games Track Athletes - All

WARMUP:
Instructor Lead
30/20/30
Then
Barbell Skills Complex w/Bar
5 Rounds of
DL: 3
CL: 3
FSQ: 3
PJ: 3
OHS: 3
PSN: 3

EQUIPMENT:
BB 225/#155;
BB #135/#95

WOD:
DL: 12
PJ: 10
5 Rounds for time

LIFTING/SKILL DEV:
Instructor lead roll/stretch

POWER HOUR:
Zercher Squat: 5-5-5-5-5
@80% of 1RM
HSPU 5-5-5-5-5 (Strict)
Sprint: 100yds - Rest 1:00 -
10 Rounds

WEEK 5 -
TUE AUG 30 2011

PHASE I:
Games Track Athletes - All

WARMUP:
Instructor Lead
30/20/30
Then 3 Rounds of
Cindy

EQUIPMENT:
KB: 24kg/16kg;
Dynamax #20/#14

WOD:
Russian Swing: 50
Wall Ball: 20
5 Rounds for time

LIFTING/SKILL DEV:
Instructor lead roll/stretch

POWER HOUR:
Sled Pull: 100yds (#135/#90)
Sled Pull Backwards: 100yds
AMRAP: 10 Minutes
Then
Farmer's Walk:
100yds - (2) 32kg KB
Run: 200
AMRAP: 10 Minutes

WEEK 5 -
WED AUG 31 2011

PHASE I:
Games Track Athletes - All

WARMUP:
Instructor Lead
30/20/30
Then w/Bar:
Barbell Complex
5 Rounds of
DL: 3
CL: 3
FSQ: 3
PP: 3
OHS: 3
PSN: 3

EQUIPMENT:
BB: #95/#65; Box: 24/20

WOD:
Push Press: 7
Box Jump: 7
Pull-Up: 7
AMRAP: 15 Minutes

LIFTING/SKILL DEV:
Instructor lead roll/stretch

POWER HOUR:
Lunge: 25yds (95/65)
Run: 50yds
AMRAP: 20 Minutes

WEEK 5 -
THU SEP 01 2011

PHASE I:
Games Track Athletes - All

WARMUP:
Instructor Lead
30/20/30
Then 3 Rounds of
Cindy

EQUIPMENT:
BB: #225/#155

WOD:
Tabata - :20/:10 x 16
DL
Burpee
Alternate between exercises -
Score each

LIFTING/SKILL DEV:
Instructor lead roll/stretch

POWER HOUR:
FSQ: Max Reps (#135/#95)
Run: 200
AMRAP: 15 Minutes

WEEK 5 -
FRI SEP 02 2011

PHASE I:
Games Track Athletes -
Rest Day

WARMUP:
Instructor Lead
30/20/30
Then w/Bar:
Barbell Complex
3 Rounds of
OHS: 3
PSNBAL: 3
HSNBAL: 3
SNBAL: 3
Then 3 Rounds of
HSN: P1: 3
HSN: P2: 3
HSN: P3: 3

EQUIPMENT:
BB + Weights

WOD:
SN: 1 EMOTM for 20 Minutes

LIFTING/SKILL DEV:
Instructor lead roll/stretch

50

WEEK 5 -
SAT SEP 03 2011

PHASE I:
Games Track Athletes - All

WARMUP:
Run: 400
30/20/30

EQUIPMENT:
BB #95/#65

WOD:
Murph

LIFTING/SKILL DEV:
Instructor lead roll/stretch

Week 6

	SUNDAY 9/4	MONDAY 9/5	TUESDAY 9/6
WARM UP	Run: 400 30/20/30		*Instructor Lead* *30/20/30* **Then 3 Rounds of** *Cindy*
EQUIPMENT	BB: 65/45 KB: (2) 32/24kg Rings		KB 24/16 DB 35/25
WOD	**A1** : Farmer's Walk: 50yds **A2** : Push Press (Score) **A3** : Ring Row (Score) *AMRAP: 15 Minutes*	*SPECIAL*	*Tabata - :20/:10 x 8 - Rest* *1:00* Swing DBPP Burpee
LIFTING/SKILL	Instructor lead roll/stretch	Instructor lead roll/stretch	Instructor lead roll/stretch

GAMES Phase I	Rest	All	All
SKILL/DEV WORK			Wall Walk: 10 Ring Support - :20/:10 x 8 Ring Bottom - :20/:10 x 8 DHPU: 3-3-3-3-3 (Strict) Dip: 5-5-5-5-5 (Strict)
GAMES WOD			Thruster: 3-3-3-3-3 (135/95)
ACCESSORY			GHD 15/15 x 5
POWER HOUR Week #1 All lifts @ 80% of 1RM		BSQ 5 x 5 Press 5 x 5 Sled Drag: 800 - #135/#90 *for time*	FSQ 5 x 5 Push Jerk 5 x 5 **Then** Butcher HiPush: 25 (135/90) Run 50 *AMRAP: 10 Minutes*

WEDNESDAY 9/7	THURSDAY 9/8	FRIDAY 9/9	SATURDAY 9/10
Instructor Lead 30/20/30 **Then 5 Rounds of** HRPU: 10 AbMat: 20	*Instructor Lead* 30/20/30 **Then 3 Rounds of** *Cindy*	*Instructor Lead* 30/20/30 **Then 5 Rounds of** HRPU: 10 AbMat: 20	**4 Rounds of** :15 Jumping Jack :15 Squat :15 MC :15 Jump Squat
BB: #135/95 *(In Rack)*	BB #135/95 AbMat	Slammer #30/#20 KB 28/20	KB 32/24
BSQ: 10 Reps *EMOTM* *for 10 Minutes* *Rest 3:00* *Then* Sprint: 25 Jog: 50 *AMRAP: 10 Minutes*	Cluster: 5 Push Up: 10 AbMat: 15 *AMRAP: 20 Minutes*	Run: 100 Ball Slam: 12 Swing: 12 *6 Rounds for time*	*Eva - 40:00 Cap*
Instructor lead roll/stretch	Instructor lead roll/stretch	Instructor lead roll/stretch	Instructor lead roll/stretch

All	All	Games Only	All
L-Sit - :20/:10 x 8 Handle Carry: 200yds #90/#70 MU Transition: 10 Rope Climb: 5 Double Under: 100	Wall Walk: 10 Ring Support - :20/:10 x 8 Ring Bottom - :20/:10 x 8 DHPU: 3-3-3-3-3 (Strict) Dip: 5-5-5-5-5 (Strict)		
Pull Up: 3 Burpee: 6 *5 Rounds for time*	CL from Blocks 3-3-3-3-3 SN from Blocks 3-3-3-3-3 *Only loads over 80% of* *1RM count as a set.*	Timed Run: 6400 Meters - *On a track. (16 laps)*	
Reverse Hyper: 30	GHD 15/15 x 3		
DL 5 x 5 Split Jerk 5 x 5 Sled Drag: 800 - #135/ #90 *for time*	OHS 5 x 5 Pull Up 5 x 5 *Then* Butcher HiPush: 25 (135/90) Run 50 *AMRAP: 10 Minutes*		

**WEEK 6 -
SUN SEP 04 2011**

PHASE I:
Games Track Athletes - Rest

WARMUP:
Run: 400
30/20/30

EQUIPMENT:
KB (2) 32/24kg; BB: 65/45;
Rings

WOD:
P1: Farmer's Walk: 50yds
P2: Push Press (Score)
P3: Ring Row (Score)
AMRAP: 15 Minutes

LIFTING/SKILL DEV:
Instructor lead roll/stretch

POWER HOUR:
Week #1

**WEEK 6 -
MON SEP 05 2011**

PHASE I:
Games Track Athletes - All

WOD:
SPECIAL

LIFTING/SKILL DEV:
Instructor lead roll/stretch

POWER HOUR:
BSQ 5 x 5 @80% of 1RM
Press 5 x 5 @80% of 1RM
Then
Sled Drag: 800 - #135/#90
For time

WEEK 6 -
TUES SEP 06 2011

PHASE I:
Games Track Athletes - All

WARMUP:
Instructor Lead
30/20/30
Then 3 Rounds of
Cindy

EQUIPMENT:
KB 24/16; DB 35/25

WOD:
Tabata: 20/10 x 8 1:00r
Swing
DBPP
Burpee

LIFTING/SKILL DEV:
Instructor lead roll/stretch

SKILL/DEV. WORK:
Wall Walk: 10
Ring Support - :20/10 x 8
Ring Bottom - :20/10 x 8
DHPU: 3-3-3-3-3 (Strict)
Dip: 5-5-5-5-5 (Strict)

GAMES WOD:
Thruster: 3-3-3-3-3 (135/95)

ACCESSORY:
GHD 15/15 x 5

POWER HOUR:
FSQ 5 x 5 @80% of 1RM
Push Jerk 5 x 5 @80% of 1RM
Then
Butcher Hi Push: 25yds (135/90)
Run: 50
AMRAP: 10 Minutes

WEEK 6 -
WED SEP 07 2011

PHASE I:
Games Track Athletes - All

WARMUP:
Instructor Lead
30/20/30
Then 5 Rounds of
HRPU: 10
AbMat: 20

EQUIPMENT:
BB: #135/95 (In Rack)

WOD:
BSQ: 10 Reps EMOTM
for 10 Minutes
Rest 3:00
Then
Sprint: 25
Jog: 50
AMRAP: 10 Minutes

LIFTING/SKILL DEV:
Instructor lead roll/stretch

SKILL/DEV. WORK:
L-Sit - :20/:10 x 8
Handle Carry: 200yds - #90/#70
MU Transitions: 10
Rope Climb: 5
Double Under: 100

GAMES WOD:
Pull Up: 3
Burpee: 6
5 Rounds for time

ACCESSORY:
Reverse Hyper: 30

POWER HOUR:
DL 5 x 5 @80% of 1RM
Split Jerk 5 x 5 @80% of 1RM
Then Sled Drag: 800 - #135/#90
For time

55

WEEK 6 -
THU SEPT 08 2011

PHASE I:
Games Track Athletes - All

WARMUP:
Instructor Lead
30/20/30
Then 3 Rounds of
Cindy

EQUIPMENT:
BB #135/95; AbMat

WOD:
Cluster: 5
Push Up: 10
AbMat: 15
AMRAP: 20 Minutes

LIFTING/SKILL DEV:
Instructor lead roll/stretch

SKILL/DEV. WORK:
Wall Walk: 10
Ring Support - :20/:10 x 8
Ring Bottom - :20/:10 x 8
DHPU: 3-3-3-3-3
Dip: 5-5-5-5-5

GAMES WOD:
CL from Blocks 3-3-3-3-3
SN from Blocks 3-3-3-3-3
Only loads over 80% of
1RM count as a set

ACCESSORY:
GHD 15/15 x 3

POWER HOUR:
OHS 5 x 5 @80% of 1RM
Pull Up 5 x 5 (Strict)
Then
Butcher Hi Push: 25yds (135/90)
Run 50
AMRAP: 10 Minutes

WEEK 6 -
FRI SEP 09 2011

PHASE I:
Games Track Athletes -
Games Only

WARMUP:
Instructor Lead
30/20/30
Then 5 Rounds of
HRPU: 10
AbMat: 20

EQUIPMENT:
Slammer #30/#20; KB 28/20

WOD:
Run: 100
Ball Slam: 12
Russian Swing: 12
6 Rounds for time

LIFTING/SKILL DEV:
Instructor lead roll/stretch

GAMES WOD:
Timed Run: 6400 Meters -
On a track. (16 laps)

WEEK 6 -
SAT SEP 10 2011

PHASE I:
Games Track Athletes - All

WARMUP:
4 Rounds of
:15 Jumping Jack
:15 Squat
:15 MC
:15 Jump Squat

EQUIPMENT: KB 32/24

WOD:
Eva - 40:00 Cap

LIFTING/SKILL DEV:
Instructor lead roll/stretch

Week 7

	SUNDAY 9/11	MONDAY 9/12	TUESDAY 9/13
WARM UP	**4 Rounds of** :15 Jumping Jack :15 Squat :15 Mountain Climber :15 Jump Squat	*Instructor Lead* 30/20/30 **Then 3 Rounds of** KB* H2H Swing: 10 KB Snatch 5/5 KB Thruster 5/5 AbMat: 20 **Light KB*	*Instructor Lead* 30/20/30 **Then 3 Rounds of** *Cindy*
EQUIPMENT	KB: 2 x 24/16 Slammer #30/#20 DB #35/#25	Barbell #135/#95 Dynamax: #20/#14	Slammer #30/#20 Box 24/20
W O D	**A1** : KB Rack Walk 50yds **A2** : Ball Slam (Score) **A3** : Thruster (Score) *AMRAP: 15 Minutes*	Wall Ball: 50 Clean and Jerk: 10 *3 Rounds for time*	Run: 800 Slam: 15 Box Jump: 15 *3 Rounds for time*
LIFTING/SKILL	Instructor lead roll/stretch	*5 Rounds of* Power Snatch (From Blocks): 5 Rope Climb: 1	*5 Rounds of* AbMat: 30 Run: 100
GAMES **Phase I**	Rest	All	All
SKILL/DEV **WORK**		Wall Walk: 10 Ring Support - :20/:10 x 8 Ring Bottom - :20/:10 x 8 DHPU: 3-3-3-3-3 Dip: 5-5-5-5-5	L-Sit - :20/:10 x 8 Handle Carry: 200yds - 90/70 MU Transition: 10 Rope Climb: 5 Double Under: 100
ACCESSORY		GHD 15/15 x 3	Reverse Hyper: 15 x 3
POWER HOUR **All lifts @ 90%** **of 1RM**		FSQ 3-3-3-3-3 Push Jerk 3-3-3-3-3 **Then** Butcher HiPush: 25 (135/90) Run 50 *AMRAP: 10 Minutes*	DL 3-3-3-3-3 Split Jerk 3-3-3-3-3 Sled Drag: 800 - #135/ #90 *for time*

WEDNESDAY 9/14	THURSDAY 9/15	FRIDAY 9/16	SATURDAY 9/17
Instructor Lead 30/20/30 **Then 3 Rounds of** KB H2H Swing: 10 KB Snatch 5/5 KB Thruster 5/5 AbMat: 20	*Instructor Lead* 30/20/30 **Then 3 Rounds of** *Cindy*	*Instructor Lead* 30/20/30 **Then 3 Rounds of** KB H2H Swing: 10 KB Snatch 5/5 KB Thruster 5/5 AbMat: 20	**4 Rounds of** :15 Jumping Jack :15 Squat :15 Mountain Climber :15 Jump Squat
BB #95/#65	BB 95/65	KB 24/16 Dynamax #20/#14	
Push Press: 12 BSQ: 20 *5 Rounds for time*	Snatch Pull Up *21, 15, 9 for time*	American Swing: 15 Wall Ball: 15 *4 Rounds for time*	*FGB*
5 Rounds of PCL from Blocks: 5 Rope Climb: 1	*3 Rounds of* Good Morning/Squat: 10 (95/65) T2B: 10	Instructor lead roll/stretch	

All	All	Rest	All
Wall Walk: 10 Ring Support - :20/:10 x 8 Ring Bottom - :20/:10 x 8 DHPU: 3-3-3-3-3 Dip: 5-5-5-5-5	L-Sit - :20/:10 x 8 Handle Carry: 200yds - 90/70 MU Transition: 10 Rope Climb: 5 Double Under: 100		
GHD 15/15 x 3	Reverse Hyper: 15 x 3		
OHS 3-3-3-3-3 Pull Up 3-3-3-3-3 (Strict) **Then** Butcher HiPush: 25 (135/90) Run 50 *AMRAP: 10 Minutes*	BSQ 3-3-3-3-3 Press 3-3-3-3-3 **Then** Sled Drag: 800 - #135/ #90 *for time*		

WEEK 7 -
SUN SEP 11 2011

PHASE I:
Games Track Athletes - Rest Day

WARMUP:
4 Rounds of
:15 Jumping Jack
:15 Squat
:15 Mountain Climber
:15 Jump Squat

EQUIPMENT:
KB: 2x 24/16;
Slammer #30/#20;
DB #35/#25

WOD:
P1: KB Rack Walk 50yds
P2: Ball Slam: Score
P3: Thruster: Score
AMRAP: 15 Minutes

LIFTING/SKILL DEV:
Instructor lead roll/stretch

WEEK 7 -
MON SEP 12 2011

PHASE I:
Games Track Athletes - All

WARMUP:
Instructor Lead
30/20/30
Then 3 Rounds of
KB* H2H Swing: 10
KB Snatch 5/5
KB Thruster 5/5
AbMat: 20
*Light KB

EQUIPMENT:
Barbell #135/#95;
Dynamax: #20/#14

WOD:
Wall Ball: 50
Clean and Jerk: 10
3 Rounds for time

LIFTING/SKILL DEV:
5 Rounds of
Power Snatch
(From Blocks): 5
Rope Climb: 1

SKILL/DEV. WORK:
Wall Walk: 10
Ring Support - :20/:10 x 8
Ring Bottom - :20/:10 x 8
DHPU 3-3-3-3-3
Dip: 5-5-5-5-5

ACCESSORY:
GHD 15/15 x 3

POWER HOUR:
FSQ 3-3-3-3-3 @90% of 1RM
Push Jerk 3-3-3-3-3
@90% of 1RM
Then
Butcher Hi Push: 25yds (135/90)
Run 50
AMRAP: 10 Minutes

WEEK 7 - TUE SEPT 13 2011

PHASE I:
Games Track Athletes - All

WARMUP:
Instructor Lead
30/20/30
Then 3 Rounds of
Cindy

EQUIPMENT:
Slammer #30/#20; Box 24/20

WOD:
Run: 800
Slam: 15
Box Jump: 15
3 Rounds for time

LIFTING/SKILL DEV:
5 Rounds of
AbMat: 30
Run: 100

SKILL/DEV. WORK:
L-Sit - :20/:10 x 8
Handle Carry: 200yds - #90/#70
MU Transitions: 10
Rope Climb: 5
Double Under: 100

ACCESSORY:
Reverse Hyper: 15 x 3

POWER HOUR:
DL 3-3-3-3-3 @90% of 1RM
Split Jerk 3-3-3-3-3
@90% of 1RM
Then
Sled Drag: 800 - #135/#90
For time

WEEK 7 - WED SEP 14 2011

PHASE I:
Games Track Athletes - All

WARMUP:
Instructor Lead
30/20/30
Then 3 Rounds of
KB H2H Swing: 10
KB Snatch 5/5
KB Thruster 5/5
AbMat: 20

EQUIPMENT: BB #95/#65

WOD:
Push Press: 12
BSQ: 20
5 Rounds for time

LIFTING/SKILL DEV:
5 Rounds of
PCL from Blocks: 5
Rope Climb: 1

SKILL/DEV. WORK:
Wall Walk: 10
Ring Support - :20/:10 x 8
Ring Bottom - :20/:10 x 8
DHPU: 3-3-3-3-3
Dip: 5-5-5-5-5

ACCESSORY:
GHD 15/15 x 3

POWER HOUR:
OHS 3-3-3-3-3 @90% of 1RM
Pull Up 3-3-3-3-3 (Strict)
Then
Butcher Hi Push: 25yds (135/90)
Run: 50yds
AMRAP: 10 Minutes

WEEK 7 - THU SEP 15 2011

PHASE I:
Games Track Athletes - All

WARMUP:
Instructor Lead
30/20/30
Then 3 Rounds of
Cindy

EQUIPMENT: BB 95/65

WOD:
Snatch
Pull Up
21, 15, 9 for time

LIFTING/SKILL DEV:
3 Rounds of
Good Morning/Squat: 10
(95/65)
T2B: 10

SKILL/DEV. WORK:
L-Sit - :20/:10 x 8
Handle Carry: 200yds - 90/70
MU Transitions: 10
Rope Climb: 5
Double Under: 100

ACCESSORY:
Reverse Hyper: 15 x 3

POWER HOUR:
BSQ 3-3-3-3-3 @90% of 1RM
Press 3-3-3-3-3 @90% of 1RM
Then
Sled Drag: 800 - #135/#90
For time

WEEK 7 - FRI SEP 16 2011

PHASE I:
Games Track Athletes -
Rest Day

WARMUP:
Instructor Lead
30/20/30
Then 3 Rounds of
KB H2H Swing: 10
KB Snatch 5/5
KB Thruster 5/5
AbMat: 20

EQUIPMENT:
KB 24/16; Dynamax
#20/#14

WOD:
American Swing: 15
Wall Ball: 15
4 Rounds for time

LIFTING/SKILL DEV:
Instructor lead roll/stretch

WEEK 7 -
SAT SEP 17 2011

PHASE I:
Games Track Athletes - All

WARMUP:
4 Rounds of
:15 Jumping Jack
:15 Squat
:15 Mountain Climber
:15 Jump Squat

EQUIPMENT: BB #95/#65

WOD:
FGB

LIFTING/SKILL DEV:
Instructor lead roll/stretch

Week 8

	SUNDAY 9/18	MONDAY 9/19	TUESDAY 9/20
WARM UP	Run: 400 30/20/30 **Then 4 Rounds of** :15 Jumping Jack :15 Squat :15 MC :15 Jump Squat	*Instructor Lead* 30/20/30 **Then 3 Rounds of** KB* H2H Swing: 10 KB Snatch 5/5 KB Thruster 5/5 AbMat: 20 *Light KB*	*Instructor Lead* 30/20/30 **Then 3 Rounds of** *Cindy*
EQUIPMENT	Handle: 90/70 KB: 32/24 Slammer #30/#20	BB: #135/#95	Box: 24/20
WOD	**A1** : Handle Carry: 50 **A2** : Swing (Score) **A3** : Slam (Score) *AMRAP: 12* *Minutes*	Run: 400 BSQ: 20 *3 Rounds for time*	Row: 1000 *Then* Box Jump: 21 Pull Up: 15 Burpee: 9 *3 Rounds for time*
LIFTING/SKILL	Instructor lead roll/stretch	Clean from blocks: 3-3-3-3-3 (80%+ of 1RM)	Snatch from blocks: 3-3-3-3-3 (80%+ of 1RM)

GAMES Phase I	Rest	All	All
SKILL/DEV WORK		L-Sit - :20/:10 x 8 Handle Carry: 200yds - #90/#70 MU Transition: 10 Rope Climb: 5 Double Under: 100	Wall Walk: 10 Ring Support -:20/10 x 8 Ring Bottom - :20/10 x 8 DHPU: 3-3-3-3-3 Dip: 5-5-5-5-5
ACCESSORY		GHD 15/15 x 3	Reverse Hyper: 15 x 3
POWER HOUR **All lifts** **Establish** **1 Rep Max**		DL 1-1-1-1-1-1-1 Split Jerk 1-1-1-1-1-1-1 Sled Drag: 800 - #135/ #90 *for time*	OHS 1-1-1-1-1-1-1 Pull Up 1-1-1-1-1-1-1 (Strict) **Then** Butcher HiPush: 25 (135/90) Run 50 *AMRAP: 10 Minutes*

WEDNESDAY 9/21	THURSDAY 9/22	FRIDAY 9/23	SATURDAY 9/24
Instructor Lead	*Instructor Lead*	*Instructor Lead*	30/20/30
30/20/30	30/20/30	30/20/30	**Then**
Then 3 Rounds of	**Then 3 Rounds of**	**Then 3 Rounds of**	:15 Jumping Jack
KB H2H Swing: 10	*Cindy*	KB H2H Swing: 10	:15 Squat
KB Snatch 5/5		KB Snatch 5/5	:15 Mountain Climber
KB Thruster 5/5		KB Thruster 5/5	:15 Jump Squat
AbMat: 20		AbMat: 20	
BB: 135/95	KB: 24/16	DB 35/25	BB #135/95
		Box 24/20	BB #245/165
		Slammer #30/20	KB 32/24
Run: 400	Swing: 20	Push Press: 21	*The Seven:*
FSQ: 12 (No Rack)	Dip: 10	Box Jump: 21	*7 Rounds of*
Ring Push Up: 12	*7 Rounds for time*	Ball Slam: 15	HSPU: 7
3 Rounds for time		Push Up: 15	Thruster: 7
		Pull Up: 9	K2E: 7
		Burpee: 9	DL: 7
		3 Rounds for time	Burpee: 7
			American Swing: 7
			Pull Up: 7
Instructor lead roll/stretch	Instructor lead roll/stretch	Instructor lead roll/stretch	Instructor lead roll/stretch

All	All	Rest	All
L-Sit - :20/:10 x 8	Wall Walk: 10		
Handle Carry:	Ring Support - :20/10 x 8		
200yds - #90/#70	Ring Bottom - :20/10 x 8		
MU Transition: 10	DHPU: 3-3-3-3-3		
Rope Climb: 5	Dip: 5-5-5-5-5		
Double Under: 100			
GHD 15/15/ x 3	Reverse Hyper: 15 x 3		
BSQ 1-1-1-1-1-1-1	FSQ 1-1-1-1-1-1-1		
Press 1-1-1-1-1-1-1	Push Jerk 1-1-1-1-1-1-1		
Then	**Then**		
Sled Drag: 800 -	Butcher HiPush: 25 (135/90)		
#135/#90 *for time*	Run 50		
	AMRAP: 10 Minutes		

65

WEEK 8 - SUN SEP 18 2011

PHASE I:
Games Track Athletes - Rest

WARMUP:
Run: 400
30/20/30
Then 4 Rounds of
:15 Jumping Jack
:15 Squat
:15 Mountain Climber
:15 Jump Squat

EQUIPMENT:
Handle: #90/#70;
KB: 32/24; Slammer #30/#20

WOD:
P1: Handle Carry: 50yds
P2: Swing (Score)
P3: Slam (Score)
AMRAP: 12 Minutes

LIFTING/SKILL DEV:
Instructor lead roll/stretch

WEEK 8 - MON SEP 19 2011

PHASE I:
Games Track Athletes - All

WARMUP:
Instructor Lead
30/20/30
Then 3 Rounds of
KB* H2H Swing: 10
KB Snatch 5/5
KB Thruster 5/5
AbMat: 20
*Light KB

EQUIPMENT: BB: #135/#95

WOD:
Run: 400
BSQ: 20
3 Rounds for time

LIFTING/SKILL DEV:
Clean from blocks: 3-3-3-3-3
(80%+ of 1RM)

SKILL/DEV. WORK:
L-Sit - :20/:10 x 8
Handle Carry: 200yds - #90/#70
MU Transitions: 10
Rope Climb: 5
Double Under: 100

ACCESSORY:
GHD 15/15 x 3

POWER HOUR:
DL 1-1-1-1-1-1-1
Establish 1 Rep Max
Split Jerk 1-1-1-1-1-1-1
Establish 1 Rep Max
Then
Sled Drag: 800 - #135/#90
For time

WEEK 8 -
TUE SEP 20 2011

PHASE I:
Games Track Athletes - All

WARMUP:
Instructor Lead
30/20/30
Then 3 Rounds of
Cindy

EQUIPMENT: Box: 24/20
WOD:
Row: 1000
Then
Box Jump: 21
Pull Up: 15
Burpee: 9
3 Rounds for time

LIFTING/SKILL DEV:
Snatch from blocks:
3-3-3-3-3 (80%+ of 1RM)

SKILL/DEV. WORK:
Wall Walk: 10
Ring Support - :20/10 x 8
Ring Bottom - :20/10 x 8
DHPU: 3-3-3-3-3
Dip: 5-5-5-5-5

ACCESSORY:
Reverse Hyper: 15 x 3

POWER HOUR:
OHS 1-1-1-1-1-1-1
Establish 1 Rep Max
Pull Up 1-1-1-1-1-1-1 (Strict)
Then
Butcher Hi Push: 25yds
(135/90)
Run 50
AMRAP: 10 Minutes

WEEK 8 -
WED SEP 21 2011

PHASE I:
Games Track Athletes - All

WARMUP:
Instructor Lead
30/20/30
Then 3 Rounds of
KB H2H Swing: 10
KB Snatch 5/5
KB Thruster 5/5
AbMat: 20

EQUIPMENT: BB: 135/95

WOD:
Run: 400
FSQ: 12 (No Rack)
Ring Push Up: 12
3 Rounds for time

LIFTING/SKILL DEV:
Instructor lead roll/stretch

SKILL/DEV. WORK:
L-Sit - :20/:10 x 8
Handle Carry: 200yds - #90/#70
MU Transitions: 10
Rope Climb: 5
Double Under: 100

ACCESSORY:
GHD 15/15 x 3

POWER HOUR:
BSQ 1-1-1-1-1-1-1
Establish 1 Rep Max
Press 1-1-1-1-1-1-1
Establish 1 Rep Max
Then
Sled Drag: 800 - #135/#90
For time

WEEK 8 - THU SEP 22 2011

PHASE I:
Games Track Athletes - All

WARMUP:
Instructor Lead
30/20/30
Then 3 Rounds of
Cindy

EQUIPMENT: KB: 24/16

WOD:
Swing: 20
Dip: 10
7 Rounds for time

LIFTING/SKILL DEV:
Instructor lead roll/stretch

SKILL/DEV. WORK:
Wall Walk: 10
Ring Support - :20/10 x 8
Ring Bottom - :20/10 x 8
DHPU: 3-3-3-3-3
Dip: 5-5-5-5-5

ACCESSORY:
Reverse Hyper: 15 x 3

POWER HOUR:
FSQ 1-1-1-1-1-1-1
Establish 1 Rep Max
Push Jerk 1-1-1-1-1-1-1
Establish 1 Rep Max
Then
Butcher Hi Push: 25yds (135/90)
Run 50yds
AMRAP: 10 Minutes

WEEK 8 - FRI SEP 23 2011

PHASE I:
Games Track Athletes - Rest

WARMUP:
Instructor Lead
30/20/30
Then 3 Rounds of
KB H2H Swing: 10
KB Snatch 5/5
KB Thruster 5/5
AbMat: 20

EQUIPMENT:
DB 35/25; Box 24/20;
Slammer #30/20

WOD:
Push Press: 21
Box Jump: 21
Ball Slam: 15
Push Up: 15
Pull Up: 9
Burpee: 9
3 Rounds for time

LIFTING/SKILL DEV:
Instructor lead roll/stretch

WEEK 8 -
SAT SEP 24 2011

PHASE I:
Games Track Athletes - All

WARMUP:
30/20/30
Then 4 Rounds of
:15 Jumping Jack
:15 Squat
:15 Mountain Climber
:15 Jump Squat

EQUIPMENT:
BB #135/95; BB #245/165;
KB 32/24

WOD:
The Seven:
HSPU: 7
Thruster: 7
K2E: 7
DL: 7
Burpee: 7
American Swing: 7
Pull Up: 7
7 Rounds

LIFTING/SKILL DEV:
Instructor lead roll/stretch

Week 9

	SUNDAY 9/25	MONDAY 9/26	TUESDAY 9/27
WARM UP	Run: 400 30/20/30	30/20/30 **Then** *Instructor Lead* **3 Rounds of** H2H Swing: 10 Snatch 5/5 Thruster 5/5 AbMat: 20	30/20/30 **Then** *Instructor Lead* **3 Rounds of** *Cindy*
EQUIPMENT	Ball #30/#20 Box 24/20 KB 28kg/20kg BB #65/#45	C2 Dynamax DB (2) #35	BB 135/95
WOD	*Tabata:* - :20/:10 x 8 - Rest 1:00 Ball Slam Burpee Box Jump American Swing Thruster	Row: 500 Squat: 40 Sit Up: 30 Push Up: 20 Pull Up: 10 *For time*	Push Press: 5 HR Push Up: 10 Ring Row: 15 *AMRAP: 20 Minutes*
LIFTING/SKILL	Instructor lead roll/stretch	Instructor lead roll/stretch	Instructor lead roll/stretch

GAMES Phase I	Rest	All	All
POWER HOUR		Zercher Squat: 5-5-5-5-5 *EMOTM* Swing 10-10-10-10-10 #124/ #88 **Then** Butcher LoPush: 25 - #90/70 Run: 50 *AMRAP: 10 Minutes*	BSQ: 5-5-5-5-5 *EMOTM* #185/#135 CL from Blocks 3-3-3-3-3 *EMOTM* Sled Pull Backwards: 800 - #135/90

WEDNESDAY 9/28	THURSDAY 9/29	FRIDAY 9/30	SATURDAY 10/1
30/20/30 **Then** *Instructor Lead* **3 Rounds of** H2H Swing: 10 Snatch 5/5 Thruster 5/5 AbMat: 20	30/20/30 **Then** *Instructor Lead* **3 Rounds of** *Cindy*	30/20/30 **Then** *Instructor Lead* **3 Rounds of** H2H Swing: 10 Snatch 5/5 Thruster 5/5 AbMat: 20	
BB #135/#95		Dynamax #20/#14	
Run: 200 DL: 15 BSQ: 10 *5 Rounds for time*	Run: 100 Pull Up: 10 Squat: 20 *10 Rounds for time*	*Karen*	*TBA*
Instructor lead roll/stretch	Instructor lead roll/stretch	Instructor lead roll/stretch	Instructor lead roll/stretch
All	**All**	**Rest**	**All**
Swing 10-10-10-10-10 #124/#88 **Then** Lunge 25 Yards (#95/#65) Run: 50 Yards *AMRAP: 20 Minutes*	FSQ 3-3-3-3-3 *EMOTM* #185/#135 SN from Blocks 3-3-3-3-3 *EMOTM* **Then** Sprint: 100 Jog: 100 *AMRAP: 10 Minutes*		

WEEK 9 -
SUN SEP 25 2011

PHASE I:
Games Track Athletes - Rest

WARMUP:
Run: 400
30/20/30

EQUIPMENT:
Ball #30/#20; Box 24/20;
KB 28kg/20kg; BB #65/#45

WOD:
Tabata: :20/:10 x 8 -
1:00 Rest
Ball Slam
Burpee
Box Jump
American Swing
Thruster

LIFTING/SKILL DEV:
Instructor lead roll/stretch

WEEK 9 -
MON SEP 26 2011

PHASE I:
Games Track Athletes - All

WARMUP:
30/20/30
Then Instructor Lead
3 Rounds of
H2H Swing: 10
Snatch: 5/5
Thruster 5/5
AbMat: 20

EQUIPMENT:
C2; Dynamax; DB (2) #35

WOD:
Row: 500
Squat: 40
Sit Up: 30
Push Up: 20
Pull Up: 10
For time

LIFTING/SKILL DEV:
Instructor lead roll/stretch

POWER HOUR:
Zercher Squat: 5-5-5-5-5
EMOTM
Swing: 10-10-10-10-10
(#124/#88)
Then
Butcher LOW push: 25 -
#90/70
Run: 50
AMRAP: 10 Minutes

WEEK 9 -
TUE SEP 27 2011

PHASE I:
Games Track Athletes - All

WARMUP:
30/20/30
Then Instructor Lead
3 Rounds of
Cindy

EQUIPMENT: BB 135/95

WOD:
Push Press: 5
Push Up: 10 (Hand Release)
Ring Row: 15
AMRAP: 20 Minutes

LIFTING/SKILL DEV:
Instructor lead roll/stretch

POWER HOUR:
BSQ: 5-5-5-5-5 EMOTM
- #185/#135
CL from Blocks:
3-3-3-3-3 EMOTM
Sled Pull: 800 BACKWARDS
- #135/90

WEEK 9 -
WED SEP 28 2011

PHASE I:
Games Track Athletes - All

WARMUP:
30/20/30
Then Instructor Lead
3 Rounds of
H2H Swing: 10
Snatch: 5/5
Thruster: 5/5
AbMat: 20

EQUIPMENT: BB #135/#95

WOD:
Run: 200
DL: 15
BSQ: 10
5 Rounds for time

LIFTING/SKILL DEV:
Instructor lead roll/stretch

POWER HOUR:
Swing: 10-10-10-10-10 (#124/#88)
Then
Lunge: 25yds (#95/#65)
Run: 50yds
AMRAP: 20 Minute

WEEK 9 -
THU SEP 29 2011

PHASE I:
Games Track Athletes - All

WARMUP:
30/20/30
Then Instructor Lead
3 Rounds of
Cindy

WOD:
Run: 100
Pull Up: 10
Squat: 20
10 Rounds for time

LIFTING/SKILL DEV:
Instructor lead roll/stretch

POWER HOUR:
FSQ 3-3-3-3-3 EMOTM
SN from Blocks 3-3-3-3-3
EMOTM #185/#135
Then
Sprint: 100
Jog: 100
AMRAP: 10 Minutes

WEEK 9 -
FRI SEP 30 2011

PHASE I:
Games Track Athletes - Rest

WARMUP:
30/20/30
Then Instructor Lead
3 Rounds of
H2H Swing: 10
Snatch 5/5
Thruster 5/5
AbMat: 20

EQUIPMENT:
Dynamax #20/#14

WOD:
Karen

LIFTING/SKILL DEV:
Instructor lead roll/stretch

WEEK 9 -
SAT OCT 1 2011

PHASE I:
Games Track Athletes - All

WOD:
TBA

LIFTING/SKILL DEV:
Instructor lead roll/stretch

Week 10

	SUNDAY 10/2	MONDAY 10/3	TUESDAY 10/4
WARM UP	:15 Jumping Jack :15 Squat :15 Mountain Climber :15 Jump Squat 30/20/30	30/20/30 **Then w/empty barbell:** **Barbell Complex** **3 Rounds of** MSCL: 3 *(From shin)* MSCL to FSQ: 3 CL: 3 Jerk: 3	30/20/30 **Then 3 Rounds of** Swing: 10 H2H Clean: 5/5 H2H Snatch 5/5 Push Up: 10
EQUIPMENT	Box 24/20	BB #135/#95	KB 24/16 Slammer #30/#20
W O D	**A1** : Run: 200 **A2** : Box Jump (Score) **A3** : Push Up (Score) *AMRAP: 12 Minutes*	Clean and Jerk (Squat): 30 *for time*	American Swing Slam Burpee *21, 15, 9 for time*
LIFTING/SKILL	Run: 25 Lunge: 25 *AMRAP: 10 Minutes*	BSQ 5-5-5-5-5 *EMOTM @80% of 1RM*	FSQ 5-5-5-5-5 *EMOTM @80% of 1RM*
GAMES Phase I	Rest	All	All
SKILL/DEV WORK		Rope Climb 1-1-1-1-1	MU (Strict): 10
ACCESSORY		GHD 15/15 x 3	Wall Walk: 10
POWER HOUR All lifts @80% of 1RM Week #1- If class is done, skip first macro lift		BSQ 5-5-5-5-5 *EMOTM* Press 5-5-5-5-5 *EMOTM* **Then** Sandbag Carry: 100 - (70/50) Run: 200 *AMRAP: 20 Minutes*	FSQ 5-5-5-5-5 *EMOTM* Push Jerk 5-5-5-5-5 *EMOTM* **Then** Butcher HiPush: 25 (140/90) Run 50 *AMRAP: 10 Minutes*

76

WEDNESDAY 10/5	THURSDAY 10/6	FRIDAY 10/7	SATURDAY 10/8
Row: 1000 30/20/30	:15 Jumping Jack :15 Squat :15 Mountain Climber :15 Jump Squat 30/20/30	30/20/30 **Then 3 Rounds of** Swing: 10 H2H Clean: 5/5 H2H Snatch 5/5 Push Up: 10	30/20/30 **Then 5 Rounds of** MSSN *(From shin)* OHS HSN - *Mid Thigh*
Dynamax #20/#14	BB 95/65	Sandbag 70/50 KB (2) 24/16	BB #135/#95
Wall: 15 Run: 200 *AMRAP: 10 Minutes*	Push Press: 12 FSQ: 15 *7 Rounds for time*	SandBag Run: 100 Farmers Walk: 100 Run: 100 *AMRAP: 20 Minutes*	*Isabel (Squat)*
DL 5-5-5-5-5-5 *EMOTM @80% of 1RM*	OHS 5-5-5-5-5 *EMOTM @80% of 1RM*		*Team Butcher Race*
All	**Rest**	**Rest**	**All**
O-Lifting Class	Double Unders: 100		
	HSPU: 3-3-3-3-3		
DL 5-5-5-5-5-5 *EMOTM* Split Jerk 5-5-5-5-5 *EMOTM* Sled Drag: 800 - #140/ #90 *for time*	OHS 5-5-5-5-5 *EMOTM* Pull Up (Strict) 5-5-5-5-5 *EMOTM* **Then** Butcher LoPush: 25 (90/70) Run 50 *AMRAP: 10 Minutes*		

WEEK 10 - SUN OCT 02 2011

PHASE I:
Games Track Athletes - Rest

WARMUP:
:15 Jumping Jack
:15 Squat
:15 Mountain Climber
:15 Jump Squat
Then
30/20/30

EQUIPMENT: Box 24/20

WOD:
P1: Run: 200
P2: Box Jump (Score)
P3: Push Up (Score)
AMRAP: 12 Minutes

LIFTING/SKILL DEV:
Run: 25
Lunge: 25
AMRAP: 10 Minutes

WEEK 10 - MON OCT 03 2011

PHASE I:
Games Track Athletes - All

WARMUP:
30/20/30
Then w/empty barbell:
Barbell Complex
3 Rounds of
MSCL: 3 (from shin)
MSCL to FSQ: 3
CL: 3
Jerk: 3

EQUIPMENT: BB #135/#95

WOD:
Clean and Jerk (Squat):
30 for time

LIFTING/SKILL DEV:
BSQ 5-5-5-5-5 EMOTM
@80% of 1RM

SKILL/DEV. WORK:
Rope Climb 1-1-1-1-1

ACCESSORY:
GHD 15/15 x 3

POWER HOUR:
*NOTE - If class is done, skip
first macro lift for power hour*
BSQ 5-5-5-5-5 EMOTM
@80% of 1RM
Press 5-5-5-5-5 EMOTM
@80% of 1RM
Then
Sandbag Carry: 100 (#70/#50)
Run: 200
AMRAP: 20 Minutes

WEEK 10 - TUE OCT 04 2011

PHASE I:
Games Track Athletes - All

WARMUP:
30/20/30
Then 3 Rounds of
Swing: 10
H2H Clean: 5/5
H2H Snatch 5/5
Push Up: 10

EQUIPMENT:
KB 24/16; Slammer #30/#20

WOD:
American Swing
Slam
Burpee
21, 15, 9 for time

LIFTING/SKILL DEV:
FSQ 5-5-5-5-5 EMOTM
@80% of 1RM

SKILL/DEV. WORK:
MU (Strict): 10
(Transitions are not strict)

ACCESSORY:
Wall Walk: 10

POWER HOUR:
*NOTE - If class is done skip
first macro lift for power hour*
FSQ 5-5-5-5-5 EMOTM
@80% of 1RM
Push Jerk 5-5-5-5-5 EMOTM
@80% of 1RM
Then
Butcher Hi Push: 25yds
(#140/#90)
Run: 50yds
AMRAP: 10 Minutes

WEEK 10 - WED OCT 05 2011

PHASE I:
Games Track Athletes - All

WARMUP:
Row: 1000
30/20/30

EQUIPMENT:
Dynamax #20/#14

WOD:
Wall: 15
Run: 200yds
AMRAP: 10 Minutes

LIFTING/SKILL DEV:
DL 5-5-5-5-5-5 EMOTM
@80% of 1RM

SKILL/DEV. WORK:
O-Lifting Class
POWER HOUR:
*NOTE - If class is done skip
 first macro lift for power hour*
DL 5-5-5-5-5-5 EMOTM
@80% of 1RM
Split Jerk 5-5-5-5-5 EMOTM
@80% of 1RM
Then
Sled Drag: 800yds - #140/#90
For time

WEEK 10 - THU OCT 06 2011

PHASE I:
Games Track Athletes - Rest

WARMUP:
:15 Jumping Jack
:15 Squat
:15 Mountain Climber
:15 Jump Squat
Then
30/20/30

EQUIPMENT: BB 95/65

WOD:
Push Press: 12
FSQ: 15
7 Rounds for time

LIFTING/SKILL DEV:
OHS 5-5-5-5-5 EMOTM
@80% of 1RM

SKILL/DEV. WORK:
Double Unders: 100
ACCESSORY:
HSPU: 3-3-3-3-3

POWER HOUR:
*NOTE - If class is done skip
first macro lift for power hour*
OHS 5-5-5-5-5 EMOTM
@80% of 1RM
Pull Up 5-5-5-5-5 (Strict)
EMOTM
Then
Butcher Low Push: 25yds
(#90/#70)
Run: 50yds
AMRAP: 10 Minutes

WEEK 10 - FRI OCT 07 2011

PHASE I:
Games Track Athletes - Rest

WARMUP:
30/20/30
Then 3 Rounds of
Swing: 10
H2H Clean: 5/5
H2H Snatch 5/5
Push Up: 10

EQUIPMENT:
Sandbag 70/50; KB (2) 24/16

WOD:
SandBag Run: 100yds
Farmer's Walk: 100yds
Run: 100yds
AMRAP: 20 Minutes

WEEK 10 -
SAT OCT 08 2011

PHASE I:
Games Track Athletes - All

WARMUP:
30/20/30
Then 5 Rounds of
MSSN: (From shin)
OHS
HSN - Mid Thigh

EQUIPMENT:
BB #135/#95

WOD:
Isabel (Squat)

LIFTING/SKILL DEV:
Team Butcher Race

Week 11

	SUNDAY 10/9	MONDAY 10/10	TUESDAY 10/11
WARM UP	Run: 400 30/20/30	:15 Jumping Jack :15 Squat :15 MC :15 Jump Squat 30/20/30	30/20/30 **Then Instructor Lead** **3 Rounds of** *Cindy*
EQUIPMENT	Butcher #90/#70 DB 35/25 KB 24kg/16kg	C2 KB 24/16 BB 95/65 AbMat	BB 135/95
WOD	**A1** : Butcher HiPush: 50yds **A2** : Push Press (Score) **A3** : American Swing (Score) *AMRAP: 12 Minutes*	Row: 1000 Swing: 50 Clean: 40 AbMat: 30 Pull Up: 20 Burpee: 10 *For time*	Run: 100 Burpee: 10 *5 Rounds for time*
LIFTING/SKILL	Instructor lead roll/stretch	FSQ 3-3-3-3-3 *EMOTM* @90% of 1RM	DL 3-3-3-3-3 *EMOTM* @90% of 1RM

GAMES Phase I	Rest	All	All
SKILL/DEV WORK		Swing 10-10-10-10-10 *EMOTM* #124/#88	Swing 10-10-10-10-10 *EMOTM* #124/#88
GAMES WOD		Ring Push Up: 10-10-10-10 *EMOTM*	Double Under 100
ACCESSORY		Rope Climb 1-1-1-1-1	MU 1-1-1-1-1-1-1-1-1
POWER HOUR **All lifts @ 90%** **of 1RM** **All strength** **sets are** **EMOTM**		FSQ 3-3-3-3-3 Push Jerk 3-3-3-3-3 **Then** Butcher HiPush: 25 (140/90) Run 50 *AMRAP: 10 Minutes*	DL 3-3-3-3-3 Split Jerk 3-3-3-3-3 Sled Drag: 800 - #135/#90 *for time*

WEDNESDAY 10/12	THURSDAY 10/13	FRIDAY 10/14	SATURDAY 10/15
:15 Jumping Jack :15 Squat :15 MC :15 Jump Squat 30/20/30	30/20/30 **Then Instructor Lead** **3 Rounds of** *Cindy*	:15 Jumping Jack :15 Squat :15 MC :15 Jump Squat 30/20/30	
BB #135/#95		Dynamax #20/#14	
Thruster: 7 Ball Slam: 14 Wall Ball: 21 *4 Rounds for time*	Box Jump: 25 Pull Up: 15 *3 Rounds for time*	Sandbag Run: 100 Wall Ball: 12 Deadlift: 12 *AMRAP: 20* *Minutes*	*TBA*
OHS 3-3-3-3-3 *EMOTM* @90% of 1RM	BSQ 3-3-3-3-3 *EMOTM* @90% of 1RM	Instructor lead roll/stretch	Instructor lead roll/stretch
All	**All**	**Rest**	**All**
Swing 10-10-10-10-10 *EMOTM* #124/#88	Swing 10-10-10-10-10 *EMOTM* #124/#88		
Pistol 10R/10L x 5	HSPU 3-3-3-3-3		
Rope Climb 1-1-1-1-1	MU 1-1-1-1-1-1-1-1-1-1		
OHS 3-3-3-3-3 Pull Up 3-3-3-3-3 (Strict) **Then** Butcher HiPush: 25 (140/90) Run 50 *AMRAP: 10 Minutes*	BSQ 3-3-3-3-3 Press 3-3-3-3-3 Sled Drag: 800 - #135/#90 *for time*		

WEEK 11 -
SUN OCT 09 2011

PHASE I:
Games Track Athletes - Rest

WARMUP:
Run: 400
30/20/30

EQUIPMENT:
Butcher #90/#70;
DB 35/25; KB 24kg/16kg

WOD:
P1: Butcher: 50yds
(High Push)
P2: Push Press: (Score)
P3: American Swing (Score)

LIFTING/SKILL DEV:
Instructor lead roll/stretch

WEEK 11 -
MON OCT 10 2011

PHASE I:
Games Track Athletes - All

WARMUP:
:15 Jumping Jack
:15 Squat
:15 Mountain Climber
:15 Jump Squat
Then
30/20/30

EQUIPMENT:
C2; KB 24/16; BB 95/65; AbMat

WOD:
Row: 1000
Swing: 50
Clean: 40
AbMat: 30
Pull Up: 20
Burpee: 10
For time

LIFTING/SKILL DEV:
FSQ 3-3-3-3-3 EMOTM
@90% of 1RM

SKILL/DEV. WORK:
Swing 10-10-10-10-10 EMOTM
(#124/#88)

GAMES WOD:
Ring Push Up: 10-10-10-10
EMOTM

ACCESSORY:
Rope Climb 1-1-1-1-1

POWER HOUR:
*Note: All strength
sets are EMOTM*
FSQ 3-3-3-3-3 @90% of 1RM
Push Jerk 3-3-3-3-3 @90% of 1RM
Then
Butcher Hi Push: 25 (140/90)
Run 50
AMRAP: 10 Minutes

WEEK 11 -
TUE OCT 11 2011

PHASE I:
Games Track Athletes - All

WARMUP:
30/20/30
Then Instructor Lead
3 Rounds of
Cindy

EQUIPMENT: BB 135/95

WOD:
Run: 100
Burpee: 10
5 Rounds for time

LIFTING/SKILL DEV:
DL 3-3-3-3-3 EMOTM
@90% of 1RM

SKILL/DEV. WORK:
Swing 10-10-10-10-10
EMOTM (#124/#88)

GAMES WOD:
Double Under 100

ACCESSORY:
MU 1-1-1-1-1-1-1-1-1-1

POWER HOUR:
*Note: All strength sets
are EMOTM*
DL 3-3-3-3-3 @90% of 1RM
Split Jerk 3-3-3-3-3
@90% of 1RM
Then
Sled Drag: 800yds - #135/#90
For time

WEEK 11 -
WED OCT 12 2011

PHASE I:
Games Track Athletes - All

WARMUP:
:15 Jumping Jack
:15 Squat
:15 Mountain Climber
:15 Jump Squat
Then
30/20/30

EQUIPMENT: BB #135/#95

WOD:
Thruster: 7
Ball Slam: 14
Wall Ball: 21
4 Rounds for time

LIFTING/SKILL DEV:
OHS 3-3-3-3-3 EMOTM
@90% of 1RM

SKILL/DEV. WORK:
Swing 10-10-10-10-10 EMOTM
(#124/#88)

GAMES WOD:
Pistol 10/10 x 5

ACCESSORY:
Rope Climb 1-1-1-1-1

POWER HOUR:
*Note: All strength sets
are EMOTM*
OHS 3-3-3-3-3 @90% of 1RM
Pull Up 3-3-3-3-3 (Strict)
Then
Butcher Hi Push: 25yds
(#140/#90)
Run: 50yds
AMRAP: 10 Minutes

WEEK 11 - THU OCT 13 2011

PHASE I:
Games Track Athletes - All

WARMUP:
30/20/30
Then Instructor Lead
3 Rounds of
Cindy

WOD:
Box Jump: 25
Pull Up: 15
3 Rounds for time

LIFTING/SKILL DEV:
BSQ 3-3-3-3-3 EMOTM
@90% of 1RM

SKILL/DEV. WORK:
Swing 10-10-10-10-10
EMOTM (#124/#88)

GAMES WOD:
HSPU 3-3-3-3-3

ACCESSORY:
MU 1-1-1-1-1-1-1-1-1-1

POWER HOUR:
*Note: All strength sets
are EMOTM*
BSQ 3-3-3-3-3 @90% of 1RM
Press 3-3-3-3-3 @90% of 1RM
Then
Sled Drag: 800yds -
#135/#90
For time

WEEK 11 - FRI OCT 14 2011

PHASE I:
Games Track Athletes - Rest

WARMUP:
:15 Jumping Jack
:15 Squat
:15 Mountain Climber
:15 Jump Squat
Then
30/20/30

EQUIPMENT:
Dynamax #20/#14

WOD:
Sandbag Run: 100
Wall Ball: 12
Deadlift: 12
AMRAP: 20 Minutes

LIFTING/SKILL DEV:
Instructor lead roll/stretch

WEEK 11 -
SAT OCT 15 2011

PHASE I:
Games Track Athletes - All

WOD:
TBA

LIFTING/SKILL DEV:
Instructor lead roll/stretch

Week 12

	SUNDAY 10/16	MONDAY 10/17	TUESDAY 10/18
WARM UP	Run: 400 30/20/30	Run: 400 30/20/30	Run: 400 30/20/30
EQUIPMENT	Handle #90/#70 C2	BB: #115/#85	BB: #95/#65
WOD	**A1** : Handle Carry: 50 **A2** : Row (Score: Calories) **A3** : Burpee (Score) *AMRAP: 12 Minutes*	Snatch: 5 Burpee: 10 7 Rounds for time	Push Jerk: 12 (95/65) SDLHP: 12 5 Rounds
LIFTING/SKILL		DL 1-1-1-1-1-1-1 Establish 1RM	OHS 1-1-1-1-1-1-1 Establish 1RM

GAMES Phase I	Rest	All	All
POWER HOUR **Max Effort** **Week-** **All lifts to** **establish 1RM**		DL 1-1-1-1-1-1-1 Split Jerk 1-1-1-1-1-1-1 Sled Drag: 800 - #135/#90 for time	OHS 1-1-1-1-1-1-1 Pull Up 1-1-1-1-1-1-1 (Strict) Then Butcher HiPush: 25 (140/90) Run 50 AMRAP: 10 Minutes

NOTES

WEDNESDAY 10/19	THURSDAY 10/20	FRIDAY 10/21	SATURDAY 10/22
Run: 400 30/20/30	Run: 400 30/20/30	Run: 400 30/20/30	Run: 400 30/20/30
BB #315/#205	C2 BB: #155/#105 KB: 32kg/24kg	DB #35/#25	BB #95/#65
Deadlift: 3 (#315/205) Box Jump: 9 5 Rounds for time	Row: 1000 **Then** Clean and Jerk American Swing 15, 12, 9 for time	Run: 400 Burpee: 12 Thruster: 12	*Roy*
BSQ 1-1-1-1-1-1-1 Establish 1RM	FSQ 1-1-1-1-1-1-1 Establish 1RM		
All	**All**	**Rest**	**All**
BSQ 1-1-1-1-1-1-1 Press 1-1-1-1-1-1-1 Sled Drag: 800 - #135/#90 for time	FSQ 1-1-1-1-1-1-1 Push Jerk 1-1-1-1-1-1-1 Then Butcher HiPush: 25 (140/90) Run 50 AMRAP: 10 Minutes		

NOTES

WEEK 12 -
SUN OCT 16 2011

PHASE I:
Games Track Athletes - Rest

WARMUP:
Run: 400
30/20/30

EQUIPMENT:
Handle #90/#70; C2

WOD:
P1: Handle Carry: 50
P2: Row - Calories - (Score)
P3: Burpee (Score)

WEEK 12 -
MON OCT 17 2011

PHASE I:
Games Track Athletes - All

WARMUP:
Run: 400
30/20/30

EQUIPMENT:
BB: #115/#85

WOD:
Snatch: 5
Burpee: 10
7 Rounds for time

LIFTING/SKILL DEV:
DL 1-1-1-1-1-1-1
Establish 1RM

POWER HOUR:
NOTE: Max Effort Week
DL 1-1-1-1-1-1-1
Establish 1RM
Split Jerk 1-1-1-1-1-1-1
Establish 1RM
Then
Sled Drag: 800 - #135/#90
For time

WEEK 12 -
TUE OCT 18 2011

PHASE I:
Games Track Athletes - All

WARMUP:
Run: 400
30/20/30

EQUIPMENT:
BB: #95/#65

WOD:
5 Rounds of
Push Jerk: 12 (95/65)
SDLHP: 12

LIFTING/SKILL DEV:
OHS 1-1-1-1-1-1-1
Establish 1RM

POWER HOUR:
NOTE: Max Effort Week
OHS 1-1-1-1-1-1-1
Establish 1RM
Pull Up 1-1-1-1-1-1-1 (Strict)
Then
Butcher Hi Push: 25 (140/90)
Run 50
AMRAP: 10 Minutes

WEEK 12 -
WED OCT 19 2011

PHASE I:
Games Track Athletes - All

WARMUP:
Run: 400
30/20/30

EQUIPMENT:
BB #315/#205

WOD:
Deadlift: 3 (#315/205)
Box Jump: 9
5 Rounds for time

LIFTING/SKILL DEV:
BSQ 1-1-1-1-1-1-1
Establish 1RM

POWER HOUR:
NOTE: Max Effort Week
BSQ 1-1-1-1-1-1-1
Establish 1RM
Press 1-1-1-1-1-1-1
Establish 1RM
Then
Sled Drag: 800 - #135/#90
For time

WEEK 12 - THU OCT 21 2011

PHASE I:
Games Track Athletes - All

WARMUP:
Run: 400
30/20/30

EQUIPMENT:
C2; BB: #155/#105;
KB: 32kg/24kg

WOD:
Row: 1000
Then
Clean and Jerk
American Swing
15, 12, 9 for time

LIFTING/SKILL DEV:
FSQ 1-1-1-1-1-1-1
Establish 1RM

POWER HOUR:
NOTE: Max Effort Week
FSQ 1-1-1-1-1-1-1
Establish 1RM
Push Jerk 1-1-1-1-1-1-1
Establish 1RM
Then
Butcher Hi Push: 25 (140/90)
Run 50
AMRAP: 10 Minutes

WEEK 12 - FRI OCT 22 2011

PHASE I:
Games Track Athletes - Rest

WARMUP:
Run: 400
30/20/30

EQUIPMENT:
DB #35/#25

WOD:
Run: 400
Burpee: 12
Thruster: 12

WEEK 12 -
SAT OCT 23 2011

PHASE I:
Games Track Athletes - All

WARMUP:
Run: 400
30/20/30

EQUIPMENT:
BB #95/#65

WOD:
Roy

Week 13

	SUNDAY 10/23	MONDAY 10/24	TUESDAY 10/25
WARM UP	*Stove Pipe* **5 Rounds of** **A1** : Row 1:00 **A2** : Static KB Hold - (24/16) x 2	**4 Rounds of** :15 Jumping Jacks :15 Squat :15 Mountain Climber :15 Jump Squat	Run: 400 30/20/30
EQUIPMENT	C2 KB 24/16 Slammer #30/#20	BB #135/#95 Box 24in/20in	Dynamax #20/#14
W O D	**A1** : Row 250M **A2** : Swing (Score) **A3** : Slam (Score) *AMRAP: 15 Minutes*	*EDT - :15 x 16 - Rest 1:00 -* *3-Rep Goal* Zercher Squat PCL Burpee FSQ Box Jump	*Kandy* Pull Up: 5 Push Up: 10 Wall Ball: 15 *AMRAP: 20 Minutes*
LIFTING/SKILL	Wall Walk: 3 Box Jump: 10 (24/20) *AMRAP: 10 Minutes*	Run: 50yds Jog: 50yds *AMRAP: 10 Minutes*	Sumo Deadlift 3-3-3-3-3 Establish 3RM

GAMES Phase I	Rest	All	All
SKILL/DEV WORK		Swing 10-10-10-10-10 #124/#88	Dip 5-5-5-5-5 *(Weighted or assisted)*
GAMES Accessory		MU (Strict) 1-1-1-1-1-1-1-1-1	Rope Climb 1-1-1-1-1
POWER HOUR Conjugate Week		PSN from Blocks 3-3-3-3-3-3-3 @90% of 1RM SN from Blocks 3-3-3-3-3-3-3 @90% of 1RM	PCL from Blocks 3-3-3-3-3-3-3 @90% of 1RM *Then* Press: 1 (#135/#95) Push Press: 2 Push Jerk: 3 Swing: 10 (40kg/28kg) *AMRAP: 10 Minutes*

WEDNESDAY 10/26	THURSDAY 10/27	FRIDAY 10/28	SATURDAY 10/29
30/20/30 **Then Complex w/Bar** **4 Rounds of** DL: 3 MSCL: 3 CL: 3 PJ: 3 SP: 3	**4 Rounds of** :15 Jumping Jacks :15 Squat :15 Mountain Climber :15 Jump Squat	**4 Rounds of** :15 Jumping Jacks :15 Squat :15 Mountain Climber :15 Jump Squat	Run: 400 30/20/30
BB: #155/#105	Slammer #30/#20 Dynamax #20/#14 KB 24kg/16kg Box 24in/20in BB #95/#65	DB #35/#25	BB: #135/#95 Rings
BB Complex DL CL FSQ Jerk *AMRAP: 20 Minutes*	**Tabata**- *:20/:10 x 8 - Rest* *1:00 - Score total reps per* *exercise* Slam Wall Ball Swing Box Jump Push Press FSQ	Walking Lunge (High Carry): 20 Steps Push Press: 5 Push Jerk: 5 *AMRAP: 20 Minutes*	*Elizabeth* PCL Ring Dip *21, 15, 9 for* *time*
		Instructor Games	Row: 1k *for time*

All	All	Rest	All
Swing 10-10-10-10-10 #124/#88	Dip 5-5-5-5-5 *or assisted)*		*4-Mile Time* *Trial Run*
MU (Strict) 1-1-1-1-1-1-1-1-1	Rope Climb 1-1-1-1-1		
Drop Snatch 3-3-3-3-3-3-3 Establish 3RM Block Shrugs 3-3-3-3-3-3-3 Establish 3RM *Then* Butcher LoPush: 25yds (#90/#70) Run: 50yds *AMRAP: 10 Minutes*	Floor Row 5-5-5-5-5 Establish 5RM RDL from Plates 5-5-5-5-5 Establish 5RM Snatch Balance 3-3-3-3-3-3-3 Establish 3RM		

WEEK 13 - SUN OCT 24 2011

PHASE I:
Games Track Athletes - Rest

WARMUP:
Stove Pipe:
5 Rounds of
P1: Row 1:00
P2: Static KB Hold -
(24/16) x 2

EQUIPMENT:
C2; KB 24/16;
Slammer #30/#20

WOD:
P1: Row 250M
P2: Swing (Score)
P3: Slam (Score)
AMRAP: 15 Minutes

LIFTING/SKILL DEV:
Wall Walk: 3
Box Jump (24/20): 10
AMRAP: 10 Minutes

WEEK 13 - MON OCT 24 2011

PHASE I:
Games Track Athletes - All

WARMUP:
4 Rounds of
:15 Jumping Jacks
:15 Squat
:15 Mountain Climber
:15 Jump Squat

EQUIPMENT:
BB #135/#95; Box 24in/20in

WOD:
EDT :15 x 16 - 1:00 Rest -
3 Rep Goal
Zercher Squat
PCL
Burpee
FSQ
Box Jump

LIFTING/SKILL DEV:
Run: 50yds
Jog: 50yds
AMRAP: 10 Minutes

SKILL/DEV. WORK:
Swing 10-10-10-10-10
(#124/#88)

ACCESSORY:
MU Strict 1-1-1-1-1-1-1-1-1

POWER HOUR:
NOTE: Conjugate Week
PSN from Blocks 3-3-3-3-3-3-3
@90% of 1RM
SN from Blocks 3-3-3-3-3-3-3
@90% of 1RM

WEEK 13 - TUE OCT 25 2011

PHASE I:
Games Track Athletes - All

WARMUP:
Run: 400
30/20/30!

EQUIPMENT:
Dynamax #20/#14

WOD:
Kandy
Pull Up: 5
Push Up: 10
Wall Ball: 15
AMRAP: 20 Minutes

LIFTING/SKILL DEV:
Deadlift (Sumo) 3-3-3-3-3 (Establish 3RM)

SKILL/DEV. WORK:
Dip 5-5-5-5-5
(Weighted or assisted)

ACCESSORY:
Rope Climb 1-1-1-1-1

POWER HOUR:
NOTE: Conjugate Week
PCL from Blocks 3-3-3-3-3-3-3
@90% of 1RM
Then
Press: 1 (#135/#95)
Push Press: 2
Push Jerk: 3
Russian Swing: 10 (40kg/28kg)
AMRAP: 10 Minutes

WEEK 13 - WED OCT 25 2011

PHASE I:
Games Track Athletes - All

WARMUP:
30/20/30
Then Complex w/Bar
4 Rounds of
DL: 3
MSCL: 3
CL: 3
PJ: 3
SP: 3

EQUIPMENT: BB: #155/#105

WOD:
BB Complex:
DL
CL
FSQ
Jerk
AMRAP: 20 Minutes

SKILL/DEV. WORK:
Swing 10-10-10-10-10
(#124/#88)

ACCESSORY:
MU Strict 1-1-1-1-1-1-1-1-1

POWER HOUR:
NOTE: Conjugate Week
Drop Snatch 3-3-3-3-3-3-3
(Establish 3RM)
Block Shrugs 3-3-3-3-3-3-3
(Establish 3RM)
Then
Butcher Low Push: 25yds
(#90/#70)
Run: 50yds
AMRAP: 10 Minutes

WEEK 13 - THU OCT 27 2011

PHASE I:
Games Track Athletes - All

WARMUP:
4 Rounds of
:15 Jumping Jacks
:15 Squat
:15 Mountain Climber
:15 Jump Squat

EQUIPMENT:
Slammer #30/#20;
Dynamax #20/#14;
KB 24kg/16kg; Box 24in/20in;
BB #95/#65

WOD:
Tabata - :20/:10 x 8 - 1:00 Rest
- Score total reps per exercise
Slam
Wall Ball
Swing
Box Jump
Push Press
FSQ

SKILL/DEV. WORK:
Dip 5-5-5-5-5
(Weighted or assisted)

ACCESSORY:
Rope Climb 1-1-1-1-1

POWER HOUR:
NOTE: Conjugate Week
Floor Row 5-5-5-5-5
Establish 5RM
RDL from Plates 5-5-5-5-5
Establish 5RM
Snatch Balance 3-3-3-3-3-3-3
Establish 3RM

WEEK 13 - FRI OCT 28 2011

PHASE I:
Games Track Athletes - Rest

WARMUP:
4 Rounds of
:15 Jumping Jacks
:15 Squat
:15 Mountain Climber
:15 Jump Squat

EQUIPMENT:
DB #35/#25

WOD:
Walking Lunge -
High Carry: 20 Steps
Push Press: 5
Push Jerk: 5
AMRAP: 20 Minutes

LIFTING/SKILL DEV:
Instructor Games

WEEK 13 -
SAT OCT 29 2011

PHASE I:
Games Track Athletes - All

WARMUP:
Run: 400
30/20/30

EQUIPMENT:
BB: #135/#95; Rings

WOD:
Elizabeth:
PCL
Ring Dip
21, 15, 9 for time

LIFTING/SKILL DEV:
Row: 1k for time

SKILL/DEV. WORK:
4 Mile Time Trial Run

99

Week 14

	SUNDAY 10/30	MONDAY 10/31	TUESDAY 11/1
WARM UP	4 Rounds of :15 Jumping Jack :15 Squat :15 MC :15 Jump Squat	Run: 400 30/20/30	4 Rounds of :15 Jumping Jack :15 Squat :15 MC :15 Jump Squat
EQUIPMENT	KB: 24/16kg Slammer: #30/#20 Box: 24in/20in Dynamax: #20/14	BB + Rack	BB + Rack
WOD	Swing: 2-20 x 2 Push Up: 1-10 x 1 Ball Slam: 2-20 x 2 Box Jump: 1-10 x 1 Wall Ball: 2-20 x 2	BSQ: 5-5-5-5-5 E3M @80% of 1RM	FSQ: 5-5-5-5-5 E3M @80% of 1RM
LIFTING/SKILL		Pull Up: 7 Push Up: 14 Squat: 21 *AMRAP: 10 Minutes*	PCL: 3 (#135/#95) Push Up: 6 Air Squat: 9 *AMRAP: 3 Minutes - Rest 1:00 - 5 Rounds*

GAMES Phase I	Rest	All	All
SKILL/DEV WORK		MU Transition 5-5-5-5-5	Rope Climb 2-2-2-2-2
GAMES WOD			
ACCESSORY		Double Under: 100	HSPU (Strict) 3-3-3-3-3
POWER HOUR Week #1 All lifts @ 80% of 1RM		BSQ 5-5-5-5-5 Press 5-5-5-5-5 CL from Blocks 5-5-5-5-5	FSQ 5-5-5-5-5 Push Jerk 5-5-5-5-5 CL Pulls from Blocks 5-5-5-5-5

WEDNESDAY 11/2	THURSDAY 11/3	FRIDAY 11/4	SATURDAY 11/5
4 Rounds of :15 Jumping Jack :15 Squat :15 MC :15 Jump Squat	Run: 400 30/20/30	**4 Rounds of** :15 Jumping Jack :15 Squat :15 MC :15 Jump Squat	**4 Rounds of** :15 Jumping Jack :15 Squat :15 MC :15 Jump Squat
BB + Rack	BB + Rack	Dynamax #20/14 C2 Box 24/20	BB: 75/#55 (2) Box 20in Dynamax #20/14 C2
DL: 5-5-5-5-5 E3M @80% of 1RM	OHS: 5-5-5-5-5 E3M @80% of 1RM	**A1** : Wall Ball: 15 **A2** : Row (Score: Calories) **A3** : Box Jump (Score) *AMRAP: 15 Minutes*	***Championship*** ***FGB*** *- 5 Rounds*
Push Press: 12 (#95/65) Power Snatch: 12 Back Squat: 12 *AMRAP: 15 Minutes*	Thruster (#95/#65) Pull Up *21, 15, 9 for time - 10:00* *Time Cap*	***Instructor Play***	*Really?*
All	**All**	**Rest**	**All**
Wall Walk 2-2-2-2-2	GHD 10/10 x 5		
Double Under: 25 Burpee: 5 *4 Rounds for time*			
	Swing 10-10-10-10-10 #124/88		
DL 5-5-5-5-5 Split Jerk 5-5-5-5-5 SN from Blocks 5-5-5-5-5	OHS 5-5-5-5-5 Pull Up (Strict) 5-5-5-5-5 SN Pull from Blocks 5-5-5-5-5		

WEEK 14 -
SUN OCT 30 2011

PHASE I:
Games Track Athletes - Rest

WARMUP:
4 Rounds of
:15 Jumping Jack
:15 Squat
:15 MC
:15 Jump Squat

EQUIPMENT:
KB: 24/16kg;
Slammer: #30/#20;
Box: 24/20in;
Dynamax #20/14

WOD:
Swing: 2-20 x 2
Push Up: 1-10 x 1
Ball Slam: 2-20 x 2
Box Jump: 1-10 x 1
Wall Ball: 2-20 x 2

WEEK 14 -
MON OCT 31 2011

PHASE I:
Games Track Athletes - All

WARMUP:
Run: 400
30/20/30

EQUIPMENT:
BB + Rack

WOD:
BSQ: 5-5-5-5-5 E3M
@80% of 1RM

LIFTING/SKILL DEV:
Pull Up: 7
Push Up: 14
Squat: 21
AMRAP: 10 Minutes

SKILL/DEV. WORK:
Muscle Up Transitions
5-5-5-5-5

ACCESSORY:
Double Under: 100

POWER HOUR:
Week #1
BSQ 5-5-5-5-5
@80% of 1RM
Press 5-5-5-5-5
@80% of 1RM
CL from Blocks 5-5-5-5-5
@80% of 1RM

WEEK 14 - TUE NOV 01 2011

PHASE I:
Games Track Athletes - All

WARMUP:
4 Rounds of
:15 Jumping Jack
:15 Squat
:15 MC
:15 Jump Squat

EQUIPMENT:
BB + Rack

WOD:
FSQ: 5-5-5-5-5 E3M
@80% of 1RM

LIFTING/SKILL DEV:
PCL: 3 (#135/#95)
Push Up: 6
Air Squat: 9
AMRAP: 3:00 - 1:00 Rest -
5 Rounds

SKILL/DEV. WORK:
Rope Climb 2-2-2-2-2

ACCESSORY:
HSPU 3-3-3-3-3 (Strict)

POWER HOUR:
Week #1
FSQ 5-5-5-5-5
@80% of 1RM
Push Jerk 5-5-5-5-5
@80% of 1RM
CL Pulls from Blocks 5-5-5-5-5
@80% of 1RM

WEEK 14 - WED NOV 02 2011

PHASE I:
Games Track Athletes - All

WARMUP:
4 Rounds of
:15 Jumping Jack
:15 Squat
:15 MC
:15 Jump Squat

EQUIPMENT:
BB + Rack

WOD:
DL: 5-5-5-5-5 E3M
@80% of 1RM

LIFTING/SKILL DEV:
Push Press: 12 (#95/65)
Power Snatch: 12
Back Squat: 12
AMRAP: 15 Minutes

SKILL/DEV. WORK:
Wall Walk 2-2-2-2-2

GAMES WOD:
Double Under: 25
Burpee: 5
4 Rounds for time

POWER HOUR:
Week #1
DL 5-5-5-5-5
@80% of 1RM
Split Jerk 5-5-5-5-5
@80% of 1RM
SN from Blocks 5-5-5-5-5
@80% of 1RM

WEEK 14 -
THU NOV 03 2011

PHASE I:
Games Track Athletes - All

WARMUP:
Run: 400
30/20/30

EQUIPMENT:
BB + Rack

WOD:
OHS: 5-5-5-5-5 E3M
@80% of 1RM

LIFTING/SKILL DEV:
Thruster (#95/#65)
Pull Up
21, 15, 9 for time -
10 Minute Cap

SKILL/DEV. WORK:
GHD 10/10 x 5

ACCESSORY:
Swing 10-10-10-10-10
(#124/#88)

POWER HOUR:
Week #1
OHS 5-5-5-5-5
@80% of 1RM
Pull Up 5-5-5-5-5 (Strict)
SN Pull from Blocks 5-5-5-5-5
@80% of 1RM

WEEK 14 -
FRI NOV 04 2011

PHASE I:
Games Track Athletes - Rest

WARMUP:
4 Rounds of
:15 Jumping Jack
:15 Squat
:15 MC
:15 Jump Squat

EQUIPMENT:
Dynamax #20/14;
C2; Box 24/20

WOD:
P1: Wall Ball: 15
P2: Row Calories (Score)
P3: Box Jump (Score)
AMRAP: 15 Minutes

LIFTING/SKILL DEV:
Instructor Play

WEEK 14 -
SAT NOV 05 2011

PHASE I:
Games Track Athletes - All

WARMUP:
4 Rounds of
:15 Jumping Jack
:15 Squat
:15 MC
:15 Jump Squat

EQUIPMENT:
BB: 75/#55 (2); Box 20in;
Dynamax #20/14; C2

WOD:
Championship FGB - 5 Rounds

LIFTING/SKILL DEV:
Really?

NOTES

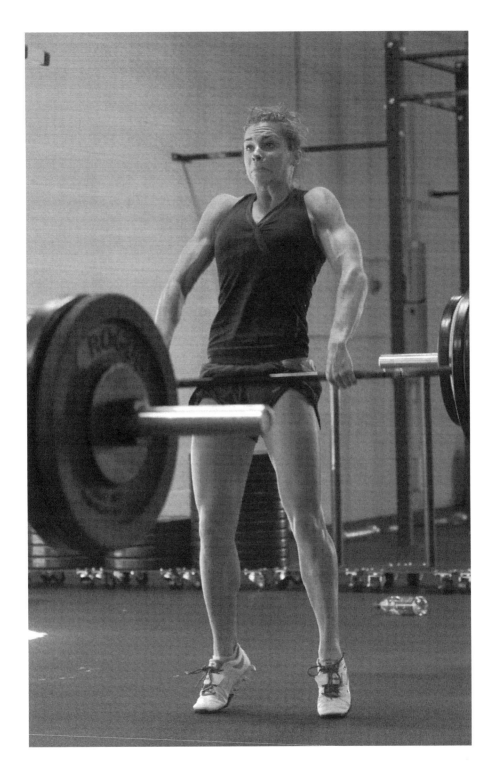

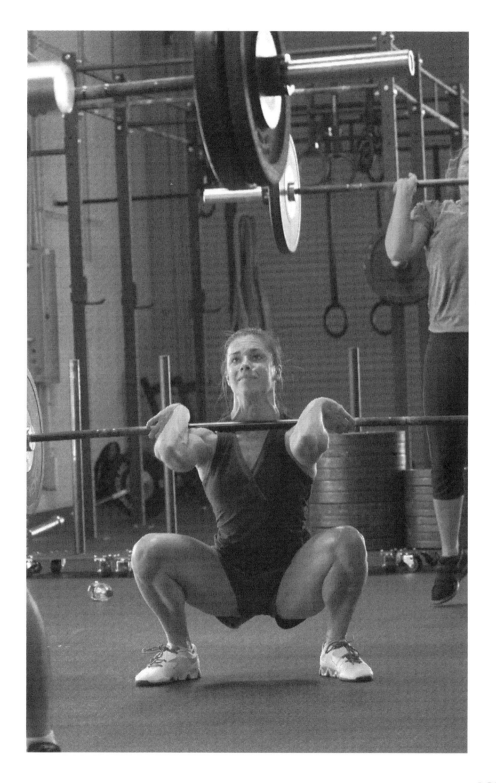

Week 15

	SUNDAY 11/6	MONDAY 11/7	TUESDAY 11/8
WARM UP	Run: 400 30/20/30 MBCL: Progression warmup - *30 Reps* *together*	**4 Rounds of** :15 Jumping Jack :15 Squat :15 MC :15 Jump Squat **Then** 30/20/30	30/20/30 **Then Instructor Lead** **3 Rounds of** *Cindy*
EQUIPMENT	Box: 24/20 Slammer 50/30 Dynamax: 20/14	BB + Rack	BB
WOD	**A1** : Box Jump: 15 **A2** : MBCL (Score) **A3** : Wall Ball(Score) *AMRAP: 12 Minutes*	FSQ 3-3-3-3-3 E3M @90% of 1RM	DL 3-3-3-3-3 E3M @90% of 1RM
LIFTING/SKILL	*Skill Development -* *Muscle Up*	Row: 1000 BSQ from Rack: 30 (225/155) *For time*	PJ: 5 (135/95) Burpee: 7 American Swing: 9 (32/24) *AMRAP: 10 Minutes*

GAMES Phase I	Rest	All	All
SKILL/DEV WORK		Swing 10-10-10-10-10 *EMOTM #124/#88*	Swing 10-10-10-10-10 *EMOTM #124/#88*
GAMES WOD		*5 Rounds of* HSPU: 3 Burpee: 6 Pull Up: 9 - *NO BUTTERFLY PU*	Double Under: 30 BSQ: 15 (135/95) *5 Rounds for time*
ACCESSORY		Rope Climb 1-1-1-1-1	MU *(strict/transitions:* *10 transitions per MU)* 1-1-1-1-1-1-1-1-1-1
POWER HOUR **All lifts are** **E3M @ 90%** **of 1RM**		FSQ 3-3-3-3-3 Push Jerk 3-3-3-3-3 SN: 3-3-3-3-3	DL 3-3-3-3-3 Split Jerk 3-3-3-3-3 Split Squat Plyometrics 5/5 x 5

WEDNESDAY 11/9	THURSDAY 11/10	FRIDAY 11/11	SATURDAY 11/12
4 Rounds of	30/20/30	**4 Rounds of**	**4 Rounds of**
:15 Jumping Jack	**Then Instructor Lead**	:15 Jumping Jack	:15 Jumping Jack
:15 Squat	**3 Rounds of**	:15 Squat	:15 Squat
:15 MC	*Cindy*	:15 MC	:15 MC
:15 Jump Squat		:15 Jump Squat	:15 Jump Squat
Then		**Then**	**Then**
30/20/30		30/20/30	30/20/30
BB + Rack	BB + Rack		
OHS 3-3-3-3-3 E3M @90% of 1RM	BSQ 3-3-3-3-3 E3M @90% of 1RM	*Mobility Warm Up:* 20 Minutes	
Wall Ball: 75 (20/14)	AbMat: 30	Push Up (HR): 12	*Manion:*
SN: 15 (135/95)	Box Jump: 20 (24/20)	Slam: 10 (30/20)	Run: 400
For time	Swing: 30 (24/16)	PCL&J: 8 (155/105)	BSQ: 29
	AMRAP: 12 Minutes	*AMRAP: 15 Minutes*	*7 Rounds for time*
All	**All**	**Rest**	**All**
Swing 10-10-10-10-10	Swing 10-10-10-10-10		
EMOTM #124/#88	*EMOTM #124/#88*		
O-Lifting Class			*O-Lifting Class*
Rope Climb 1-1-1-1-1	MU *(strict/transitions:*		
	10 transitions per MU)		
	1-1-1-1-1-1-1-1-1-1		
OHS 3-3-3-3-3	BSQ 3-3-3-3-3		
Pull Up (Strict) 3-3-3-3-3	Press 3-3-3-3-3		
Then	Sled Drag: 800 - #180/		
Butcher HiPush: 25 (180/135)	#135 *for time*		
Run 50			
AMRAP: 10 Minutes			

WEEK 15 -
SUN NOV 06 2011

PHASE I:
Games Track Athletes - Rest

WARMUP:
Run: 400
30/20/30
MBCL: Progression warmup -
30 Reps together

EQUIPMENT:
Box: 24/20; Slammer 50/30;
Dynamax: 20/14

WOD:
P1: Box Jump: 15
P2: MBCL (Score)
P3: Wall Ball(Score)
AMRAP: 12 Minutes

LIFTING/SKILL DEV:
Skill Development - Muscle Up

WEEK 15 -
MON NOV 07 2011

PHASE I:
Games Track Athletes - All

WARMUP:
4 Rounds of
:15 Jumping Jack
:15 Squat
:15 Mountain Climber
:15 Jump Squat
Then
30/20/30

EQUIPMENT: BB + Rack

WOD:
FSQ 3-3-3-3-3 E3M
@90% of 1RM

LIFTING/SKILL DEV:
Row: 1000M
BSQ: 30 From Rack (225/155)
For time

SKILL/DEV. WORK:
NOTE: IN ADDITION TO WOD
Swing 10-10-10-10-10 EMOTM
(#124/#88)

GAMES WOD:
NOTE: IN ADDITION TO WOD
HSPU: 3
Burpee: 6
Pull Up: 9
5 Rounds - NO BUTTERFLY PU

ACCESSORY:
NOTE: IN ADDITION TO WOD
Rope Climb 1-1-1-1-1

POWER HOUR:
NOTE: IN ADDITION TO WOD;
All strength sets done every 3 minutes
FSQ 3-3-3-3-3 @90% of 1RM
Push Jerk 3-3-3-3-3
@90% of 1RM
SN: 3-3-3-3-3 @90% of 1RM

WEEK 15 -
TUE NOV 08 2011

PHASE I:
Games Track Athletes - All

WARMUP:
30/20/30
Then Instructor Lead
3 Rounds of
Cindy

EQUIPMENT: BB

WOD:
DL 3-3-3-3-3 E3M
@90% of 1RM

LIFTING/SKILL DEV:
PJ: 5 (135/95)
Burpee: 7
American Swing: 9 (32kg/24kg)
AMRAP: 10 Minutes

SKILL/DEV. WORK:
Swing 10-10-10-10-10
EMOTM (#124/#88)

GAMES WOD:
Double Under: 30
BSQ: 15 (135/95)
5 Rounds for time

ACCESSORY:
MU strict or transitions -
10 transitions per MU
MU 1-1-1-1-1-1-1-1-1-1

POWER HOUR:
All strength sets done
every 3 minutes
DL 3-3-3-3-3 @90% of 1RM
Split Jerk 3-3-3-3-3
@90% of 1RM
Split Squat Plyometrics 5/5 x 5

WEEK 15 -
WED NOV 09 2011

PHASE I:
Games Track Athletes - All

WARMUP:
4 Rounds of
:15 Jumping Jack
:15 Squat
:15 Mountain Climber
:15 Jump Squat
Then
30/20/30

EQUIPMENT: BB + Rack

WOD:
OHS 3-3-3-3-3 E3M
@90% of 1RM

LIFTING/SKILL DEV:
Wall Ball: 75 (20/14)
SN: 15 (135/95)
For time
SKILL/DEV. WORK:
NOTE: IN ADDITION TO WOD
Swing 10-10-10-10-10 EMOTM
(#124/#88)

GAMES WOD:
O-Lifting Class

ACCESSORY:
Rope Climb 1-1-1-1-1

POWER HOUR:
All strength sets done
every 3 minutes
OHS 3-3-3-3-3 @90% of 1RM
Pull Up 3-3-3-3-3 (Strict)
Then
Butcher Hi Push: 25yds (180/135)
Run: 50yds
AMRAP: 10 Minutes

111

WEEK 15 - THU NOV 10 2011

PHASE I:
Games Track Athletes - All

WARMUP:
30/20/30
Then Instructor Lead
3 Rounds of
Cindy

EQUIPMENT: BB + Rack

WOD:
BSQ 3-3-3-3-3 E3M
@90% of 1RM

LIFTING/SKILL DEV:
AbMat: 30
Box Jump: 20 (24/20)
Swing: 30 (24/16)
AMRAP: 12 Minutes

SKILL/DEV. WORK:
Swing 10-10-10-10-10 EMOTM
(#124/#88)

ACCESSORY:
MU strict or transitions - 1
0 transitions per MU
MU 1-1-1-1-1-1-1-1-1-1

POWER HOUR:
*All strength sets done
every 3 minutes*
BSQ 3-3-3-3-3 @90% of 1RM
Then
Press 3-3-3-3-3 @90% of 1RM
Then
Sled Drag: 800 - #180/#135
For time

WEEK 15 - FRI NOV 11 2011

PHASE I:
Games Track Athletes -
Rest

WARMUP:
4 Rounds of
:15 Jumping Jack
:15 Squat
:15 Mountain Climber
:15 Jump Squat
Then
30/20/30

WOD:
Mobility Warm Up:
20 Minutes

LIFTING/SKILL DEV:
Push Up (HR): 12
Slam: 10 (30/20)
PCL&J: 8 (155/105)
AMRAP: 15 Minutes

WEEK 15 -
SAT NOV 12 2011

PHASE I:
Games Track Athletes - All

WARMUP:
4 Rounds of
:15 Jumping Jack
:15 Squat
:15 Mountain Climber
:15 Jump Squat
Then
30/20/30

LIFTING/SKILL DEV:
Manion:
Run: 400
BSQ: 29
7 Rounds for time

GAMES WOD:
O-Lifting Class

Week 16

	SUNDAY 11/13	MONDAY 11/14	TUESDAY 11/15
WARM UP	Run: 400 30/20/30	Run: 400 30/20/30	Run: 400 30/20/30
EQUIPMENT	BB: 95/65	BB	BB + Rack
WOD	PP: 2-20 x 2 Push Up (HR): 1-10 x 1 FSQ: 2-20 x 2 Burpee: 1-10 x 1 Thruster: 2-20 x 2	DL 1-1-1-1-1-1-1 *E3M* Establish 1RM	OHS 1-1-1-1-1-1-1 *E3M* Establish 1RM
LIFTING/SKILL	*Instructor* *Games*	*Tabata* - *:20/:10 x 8 - Rest* *1:00* Squat Toes to Bar Burpee	Lunge (High Carry): 20 Steps - #35/#25 Rowing Push Up: 10 DBHSN: 10 *AMRAP: 15 Minutes*

GAMES Phase I	Rest	All	All
POWER HOUR **Max Effort** **Week** **All lifts** **Establish 1RM**		DL 1-1-1-1-1-1-1 Split Jerk 1-1-1-1-1-1-1 Clean from block 1-1-1-1-1-1	OHS 1-1-1-1-1-1-1 Pull Up (Strict) 1-1-1-1-1-1-1 Snatch from block 1-1-1-1-1-1-1

NOTES

_____

_____

_____

_____

_____

_____

_____

WEDNESDAY 11/16	THURSDAY 11/17	FRIDAY 11/18	SATURDAY 11/19
Run: 400 30/20/30	Run: 400 30/20/30	Run: 400 30/20/30	Run: 400 30/20/30
BB + Rack	BB + Rack	BB 75/55	
BSQ 1-1-1-1-1-1-1 *E3M* Establish 1RM	FSQ 1-1-1-1-1-1-1 *E3M* Establish 1RM	Run: 400 Thruster: 21 *3 Rounds for* *time*	*Angie:* Pull Up: 100 Push Up: 100 Sit Up: 100 Squat: 100 *For time*
Wall Ball: 12 Pull Up: 10 DL: 8 (#225/#155) *AMRAP: 10 Minutes*	Row: 500 Swing: 50 (24/16) Ball Slam: 40 (#30/20) Box Jump: 30 (24/20) Pull Up: 20 Burpee: 10	*Instructor* *Games*	*Instructor* *Games*
All	**All**	**Rest**	**All**
BSQ 1-1-1-1-1-1-1 Press 1-1-1-1-1-1-1 CL&J 1-1-1-1-1-1-1	FSQ 1-1-1-1-1-1-1 Push Jerk 1-1-1-1-1-1-1 Fat Bar Clean 1-1-1-1-1-1		

NOTES

_____

_____

_____

_____

_____

_____

_____

WEEK 16 -
SUN NOV 13 2011

PHASE I:
Games Track Athletes - Rest

WARMUP:
Run: 400
30/20/30

EQUIPMENT:
BB: 95/65

WOD:
PP: 2-20 x 2
Push Up (HR): 1-10 x 1
FSQ: 2-20 x 2
Burpee: 1-10 x 1
Thruster: 2-20 x 2

LIFTING/SKILL DEV:
Instructor Games

WEEK 16 -
MON NOV 14 2011

PHASE I:
Games Track Athletes - All

WARMUP:
Run: 400
30/20/30

EQUIPMENT: BB

WOD:
DL 1-1-1-1-1-1-1 E3M
Establish 1RM

LIFTING/SKILL DEV:
Tabata - :20/:10 x 8 - 1:00 Rest
Squat
Toes to Bar
Burpee

POWER HOUR:
NOTE: Max Effort Week
DL 1-1-1-1-1-1-1
Establish 1RM
Split Jerk 1-1-1-1-1-1-1
Establish 1RM
Clean from block 1-1-1-1-1-1
Establish 1RM

WEEK 16 - TUES NOV 15 2011

PHASE I:
Games Track Athletes - All

WARMUP:
Run: 400
30/20/30

EQUIPMENT: BB + Rack

WOD:
OHS 1-1-1-1-1-1-1 E3M
Establish 1RM

LIFTING/SKILL DEV:
Lunge (High Carry): 20 Steps - #35/#25
Rowing Push Up: 10
DBHSN: 10
AMRAP: 15 Minutes

POWER HOUR:
NOTE: Max Effort Week
OHS 1-1-1-1-1-1-1
Establish 1RM
Pull Up 1-1-1-1-1-1-1 (Strict)
Snatch from block
1-1-1-1-1-1-1
Establish 1RM

WEEK 16 - WED NOV 16 2011

PHASE I:
Games Track Athletes - All

WARMUP:
Run: 400
30/20/30

EQUIPMENT: BB + Rack

WOD:
BSQ 1-1-1-1-1-1-1 E3M
Establish 1RM

LIFTING/SKILL DEV:
Wall Ball: 12
Pull Up: 10
DL: 8 (#225/#155)
AMRAP: 10 Minutes

POWER HOUR:
NOTE: Max Effort Week
BSQ 1-1-1-1-1-1-1
Establish 1RM
Press 1-1-1-1-1-1-1
Establish 1RM
CL&J 1-1-1-1-1-1-1
Establish 1RM

**WEEK 16 -
THU NOV 17 2011**

PHASE I:
Games Track Athletes - All

WARMUP:
Run: 400
30/20/30

EQUIPMENT: BB + Rack

WOD:
FSQ 1-1-1-1-1-1-1 E3M
Establish 1RM

LIFTING/SKILL DEV:
Row: 500
Swing: 50 (24/16)
Ball Slam: 40 (#30/20)
Box Jump: 30 (24/20)
Pull Up: 20
Burpee: 10

POWER HOUR:
NOTE: Max Effort Week
FSQ 1-1-1-1-1-1-1
Establish 1RM
Push Jerk 1-1-1-1-1-1-1
Establish 1RM
Fat Bar Clean 1-1-1-1-1-1
Establish 1RM

**WEEK 16 -
FRI NOV 18 2011**

PHASE I:
Games Track Athletes - Rest

WARMUP:
Run: 400
30/20/30

EQUIPMENT: BB 75/55

WOD:
Run: 400
Thruster: 21
3 Rounds for time

LIFTING/SKILL DEV:
Instructor Games

**WEEK 16 -
SAT NOV 19 2011**

PHASE I:
Games Track Athletes - All

WARMUP:
Run: 400
30/20/30

WOD:
Angie:
Pull Up: 100
Push Up: 100
Sit Up: 100
Squat: 100
For time

LIFTING/SKILL DEV:
Instructor Games

Week 17

	SUNDAY 11/20	MONDAY 11/21	TUESDAY 11/22
WARM UP	**4 Rounds of** :15 Jumping Jack :15 Squat :15 MC :15 Jump Squat **Then** 30/20/30 *Then Partner Med Ball* *4 Rounds of* Sit Up: 10 High Toss: 10	**4 Rounds of** :15 Jumping Jack :15 Squat :15 MC :15 Jump Squat **Then** 30/20/30 *Then 5 Rounds of* *DL/CL/FSQ/SJ - 3 Reps* *each*	**Partner Rows** **5 Rounds of** **A1** : Row 1:00 **A2** : Rest *Transition :15 (Switch)*
EQUIPMENT	Box 24/20	BB #185/#135	BB: 275/#155 BB: 95/65 Rings
WOD	**A1** : Sit Up: 20 **A2** : Box Jumps (Score) **A3** : Floor Press (Score) *AMRAP: 12 Minutes*	BB Complex DL: 1 CL: 1 FSQ: 1 SJ: 1 *AMRAP: 20 Minutes*	DL :15 - *Rest :45* Thruster :15 - *Rest :45* Ring Push Up :15 - *Rest :45* Burpee :15 - *Rest :45* *5 Rounds - Score each* *movement each interval*
LIFTING/SKILL	Wall Walk: 3 Burpee: 9 *5 Rounds (not timed)*	*Instructor Play*	Turkish Get Up 1R/1L - *AMRAP: 10 Minutes*
GAMES **Phase I**	Rest	All	All
SKILL/DEV **WORK**		Swing 10-10-10-10-10 #124/#88 Reverse Hyper: 20-20-20-20-20	Ring Hold Top - :20/:10 x 8 Ring Hold Bottom - :20/:10 x 8
GAMES **WOD**		GHD Sit Up: 20 BSQ: 12 (#185/#135) *5 Rounds for time*	Rope Climb Deadlift (315/205) *5, 4, 3, 2, 1 for time*
GAMES **Accessory**		MU (Strict) 1-1-1-1-1-1-1-1-1	FSQ (w/KB) 7-7-7-7-7 (2)x32/24
POWER HOUR **Conjugate** **Week**		Power Jerk (Squat) 3-3-3-3-3 *(Practice)* SDL: 3-3-3-3-3 @90% of 1RM of DL	TGU 1R/1L - *AMRAP: 10* *Minutes* BSQ 10-10-10-10-10 @75% of 1RM

WEDNESDAY 11/23	THURSDAY 11/24	FRIDAY 11/25	SATURDAY 11/26
5 Rounds of	**4 Rounds of**	**4 Rounds of**	**4 Rounds of**
Jump Rope 1:00 -	:15 Jumping Jack	:15 Jumping Jack	:15 Jumping Jack
Transition :15	:15 Squat	:15 Squat	:15 Squat
Squat Hold (w/kb) 1:00	:15 MC	:15 MC	:15 MC
- Transition :15	:15 Jump Squat	:15 Jump Squat	:15 Jump Squat
	Then	**Then**	**Then**
	30/20/30	30/20/30	30/20/30
		PSN/OHS/SNBAL	
		Skills	
Dynamax 20/14	BB: 55/45	BB: 95/65	Jump Rope
Wall Ball: 15	Thruster	PSN 7	*Annie*
Pull Up: 5	Jumping Pull Up	OHS: 7	
AMRAP: 5 Minutes -	*21, 15, 9 - 3:00 Cap -*	SNBAL: 7	
Rest 3:00 - 5 Rounds	*Rest 2:00 - 5 Rounds*	*7 Rounds for time*	
	Really?	*Instructor Play*	*Instructor Play*
All	**All**	**Rest**	**All**
Swing 10-10-10-10-10			
#124/#88			
Muscle Up: 3			
Toes to Bar: 12			
7 Rounds for time			
SN from blocks			
Clean from blocks			
Work for 30 minutes			
on each			

WEEK 17 - SUN NOV 20 2011

PHASE I:
Games Track Athletes - Rest

WARMUP:
4 Rounds of
:15 Jumping Jack
:15 Squat
:15 Mountain Climber
:15 Jump Squat
Then
30/20/30
Then Partner Med Ball
3 Rounds of
Sit Up: 10
High Toss: 10

EQUIPMENT: Box 24/20

WOD:
P1: Sit Up: 20
P2: Box Jumps (Score)
P3: Floor Press (Score)
AMRAP: 12 Minutes

LIFTING/SKILL DEV:
Wall Walk: 3
Burpee: 9
5 Rounds (not timed)

WEEK 17 - MON NOV 21 2011

PHASE I:
Games Track Athletes - All

WARMUP:
4 Rounds of
:15 Jumping Jack
:15 Squat
:15 Mountain Climber
:15 Jump Squat
Then
30/20/30
Then 5 Rounds of
DL/CL/FSQ/SJ - 3 Reps each

EQUIPMENT: BB #185/#135

WOD:
BB Complex
DL: 1
CL: 1
FSQ: 1
SJ: 1
AMRAP: 20 Minutes

LIFTING/SKILL DEV:
Instructor Play

SKILL/DEV. WORK:
Swing 10-10-10-10-10 (#124/#88)
Reverse Hyper: 20-20-20-20-20
GAMES WOD:
GHD Sit Up: 20
BSQ: 12 (#185/#135)
5 Rounds for time

ACCESSORY:
MU Strict 1-1-1-1-1-1-1-1-1

POWER HOUR:
NOTE: Conjugate Week
Power Jerk (Squat): 3-3-3-3-3
(Practice)
SDL: 3-3-3-3-3
@90% of 1RM of DL

WEEK 17 - TUE NOV 22 2011

PHASE I:
Games Track Athletes - All

WARMUP:
Partner Rows
5 Rounds of
P1: Row 1:00
P2: Rest
:15 Transition (Switch)

EQUIPMENT:
BB: #275/#155;
BB: 95/65; Rings

WOD:
:15 Deadlift
:45 Rest
:15 Thruster
:45 Rest
:15 Ring Push Up
:45 Rest
:15 Burpee
:45 Rest
5 Rounds -
Score each movement, each interval

LIFTING/SKILL DEV:
Turkish Get Up 1/1 -
AMRAP: 10 Minutes

SKILL/DEV. WORK:
Ring Hold - Top - :20/:10 x 8
Ring Hold - Bottom - :20/:10 x 8

GAMES WOD:
Rope Climb
Deadlift (315/205)
5, 4, 3, 2, 1 for time

ACCESSORY:
Double KB FSQ: 7-7-7-7-7 (32/24)

POWER HOUR:
NOTE: Conjugate Week
Turkish Get Up 1/1 -
AMRAP: 10 Minutes
BSQ 10-10-10-10-10
@75% of 1RM

WEEK 17 - WED NOV 23 2011

PHASE I:
Games Track Athletes - All

WARMUP:
5 Rounds of
Jump Rope: 1:00 -
:15 Transition
Squat Hold w/KB: 1:00 -
:15 Transition

EQUIPMENT:
Dynamax 20/14

WOD:
Wall Ball: 15
Pull Up: 5
AMRAP: 5:00 - Rest 3:00 -
5 Rounds

SKILL/DEV. WORK:
Swing 10-10-10-10-10
(#124/#88)

GAMES WOD:
Muscle Up: 3
Toes to Bar: 12
7 Rounds for time

POWER HOUR:
NOTE: Conjugate Week
SN from blocks
Clean from blocks
Work for 30 minutes on each

WEEK 17 -
THU NOV 24 2011

PHASE I:
Games Track Athletes - All

WARMUP:
4 Rounds of
:15 Jumping Jack
:15 Squat
:15 Mountain Climber
:15 Jump Squat
Then
30/20/30

EQUIPMENT:
BB: 55/45

WOD:
Thruster
Jumping Pull Up
21, 15, 9 - 3:00 Cap -
Rest 2:00 - 5 Rounds

LIFTING/SKILL DEV:
Really?

WEEK 17 -
FRI NOV 25 2011

PHASE I:
Games Track Athletes - Rest

WARMUP:
4 Rounds of
:15 Jumping Jack
:15 Squat
:15 Mountain Climber
:15 Jump Squat
Then
30/20/30
PSN/OHS/SNBAL Skills

EQUIPMENT:
BB: 95/65
WOD:
PSN: 7
OHS: 7
SNBAL: 7
7 Rounds for time

LIFTING/SKILL DEV:
Instructor Play

WEEK 17 -
SAT NOV 26 2011

PHASE I:
Games Track Athletes - All
WARMUP:
4 Rounds of
:15 Jumping Jack
:15 Squat
:15 Mountain Climber
:15 Jump Squat
Then
30/20/30

EQUIPMENT: Jump Rope

WOD:
Annie

LIFTING/SKILL DEV:
Instructor Play

Week 18

	SUNDAY 11/27	MONDAY 11/28	TUESDAY 11/29
WARM UP	**4 Rounds of** :15 Jumping Jack :15 Squat :15 MC :15 Jump Squat	Row: 500 30/20/30	**4 Rounds of** :15 Jumping Jack :15 Squat :15 MC :15 Jump Squat
EQUIPMENT	BB: 75/55	BB + Rack	BB + Rack
WOD	**A1** : Burpee: 10 **A2** : Push Press (Score) **A3** : Floor Row (Score) *AMRAP: 12 Minutes*	BSQ: 5-5-5-5-5 *E3M* @80% of 1RM	FSQ: 5-5-5-5-5 *E3M* @80% of 1RM
LIFTING/SKILL	*Instructor Play*	Squat: 50 Pull Up: 20 *4 Rounds for time*	Swing: 20 (24/16) Wall Ball: 20 (20/14) Slam: 20 (30/20) *AMRAP: 12 Minutes*
GAMES Phase I	Rest	All	All
SKILL/DEV WORK		MU Transition 5-5-5-5-5	HSPU: 3-3-3-3-3 Dip: 10-10-10-10-10
GAMES WOD		Run 800 (Woodway) - *Rest* *3:00 - 3 Rounds (total time)*	Row: 1k
Accessory		Swing 10-10-10-10-10 #124/88	Swing 10-10-10-10-10 #124/88
POWER HOUR Week #1 All lifts @80% of 1RM		BSQ 5-5-5-5-5 Press 5-5-5-5-5 CL from Blocks 5-5-5-5-5	FSQ 5-5-5-5-5 Push Jerk 5-5-5-5-5 CL Pulls from Blocks 5-5-5-5-5

NOTES

126

WEDNESDAY 11/30	THURSDAY 12/1	FRIDAY 12/2	SATURDAY 12/3
4 Rounds of :15 Jumping Jack :15 Squat :15 MC :15 Jump Squat	Row: 500 30/20/30	**4 Rounds of** :15 Jumping Jack :15 Squat :15 MC :15 Jump Squat	**4 Rounds of** :15 Jumping Jack :15 Squat :15 MC :15 Jump Squat
BB + Rack	BB + Rack	BB: 155/105	BB 135/95
DL: 5-5-5-5-5 *E3M* @80% of 1RM	OHS: 5-5-5-5-5 *E3M* @80% of 1RM	*7 Rounds of* PCL: 7 AbMat: 30	***Amanda*** MU Snatch *9, 7, 5 for time*
CL: 1 (BB 185/#135) FSQ: 2 Jerk: 1 *AMRAP: 15 Minutes*	Thruster (95/65) Ring Push Up *10, 9, 8, 7, 6, 5, 4, 3,* *2, 1*	***Instructor Play***	If NO MU: Sub 3x Pull Ups/Dips *Then* ***Instructor Play***
All	**All**	**Rest**	**All**
Double Under: 50 Ring Push Ups: 20 *3 Rounds -* *Completion*	*3 Rounds of* Cartwheel: 10yds Forward Roll 10yds Roll Back Press to Hand Stand: 10yds Hand Walk: 10yds		***O-Lifting Class***
O-Lifting Class	MU: 30 *for time*		***Death By Rope Climb***
Swing 10-10-10-10-10 #124/88	Swing 10-10-10-10-10 #124/88		
DL 5-5-5-5-5 Split Jerk 5-5-5-5-5 SN from Blocks 5-5-5-5-5	OHS 5-5-5-5-5 Pull Up 5-5-5-5-5 SN Pull from Blocks 5-5-5-5-5		

NOTES

_____

_____

_____

WEEK 18 -
SUN NOV 27 2011

PHASE I:
Games Track Athletes - Rest

WARMUP:
4 Rounds of
:15 Jumping Jack
:15 Squat
:15 Mountain Climber
:15 Jump Squat

EQUIPMENT: BB: 75/55

WOD:
P1: Burpee: 10
P2: Push Press (Score)
P3: Floor Row (Score)
AMRAP: 12 Minutes

LIFTING/SKILL DEV:
Instructor Play

WEEK 18 -
MON NOV 28 2011

PHASE I:
Games Track Athletes - All

WARMUP:
Row: 500
30/20/30

EQUIPMENT: BB + Rack

WOD:
BSQ: 5-5-5-5-5 E3M
@80% of 1RM

LIFTING/SKILL DEV:
Squat: 50
Pull Up: 20
4 Rounds for time

SKILL/DEV. WORK:
Muscle Up Transitions
5-5-5-5-5

GAMES WOD:
Run 800 (Woodway Curve) -
Rest 3:00 -
3 Rounds (Total Time)

ACCESSORY:
Swing 10-10-10-10-10
(#124/#88)

POWER HOUR:
Week #1
BSQ 5-5-5-5-5
@80% of 1RM
Press 5-5-5-5-5
@80% of 1RM
CL from Blocks 5-5-5-5-5
@80% of 1RM

128

WEEK 18 - TUES NOV 29 2011

PHASE I:
Games Track Athletes - All

WARMUP:
4 Rounds of
:15 Jumping Jack
:15 Squat
:15 MC
:15 Jump Squat

EQUIPMENT: BB + Rack

WOD:
FSQ: 5-5-5-5-5 E3M
@80% of 1RM

LIFTING/SKILL DEV:
Swing: 20 (24/16)
Wall Ball: 20 (20/14)
Slam: 20 (30/20)
AMRAP: 12 Minutes

SKILL/DEV. WORK:
HSPU: 3-3-3-3-3
Dip: 10-10-10-10-10

GAMES WOD:
Row: 1k

ACCESSORY:
Swing 10-10-10-10-10
(#124/#88)

POWER HOUR:
Week #1
FSQ 5-5-5-5-5 @80% of 1RM
Push Jerk 5-5-5-5-5
@80% of 1RM
CL Pulls from Blocks 5-5-5-5-5
@80% of 1RM

WEEK 18 - WED NOV 30 2011

PHASE I:
Games Track Athletes - All

WARMUP:
4 Rounds of
:15 Jumping Jack
:15 Squat
:15 MC
:15 Jump Squat

EQUIPMENT: BB + Rack

WOD:
DL: 5-5-5-5-5 E3M
@80% of 1RM

LIFTING/SKILL DEV:
CL: 1 (BB 185/#135)
FSQ: 2
Jerk: 1
AMRAP 15 Minutes

SKILL/DEV. WORK:
Double Under: 50
Ring Push Ups: 20
3 Rounds (Completion)

GAMES WOD:
O-Lifting Class

ACCESSORY:
Swing 10-10-10-10-10
(#124/#88)

POWER HOUR:
Week #1
DL 5-5-5-5-5 @80% of 1RM
Split Jerk 5-5-5-5-5
@80% of 1RM
SN from Blocks 5-5-5-5-5
@80% of 1RM

WEEK 18 - THU DEC 01 2011

PHASE I:
Games Track Athletes - All

WARMUP:
Row: 500
30/20/30

EQUIPMENT: BB + Rack

WOD:
OHS: 5-5-5-5-5 E3M
@80% of 1RM

LIFTING/SKILL DEV:
Thruster (95/65)
Ring Push Up
10, 9, 8, 7, 6, 5, 4, 3, 2, 1

SKILL/DEV. WORK:
3 Rounds of
Cartwheel: 10yds
Forward Roll: 10yds
Roll Back Press
to Hand Stand: 10yds
Hand Walk: 10yds

GAMES WOD:
30 Muscle Ups for time

ACCESSORY:
Swing 10-10-10-10-10
(#124/#88)

POWER HOUR:
Week #1
OHS 5-5-5-5-5 @80% of 1RM
Pull Up 5-5-5-5-5 (Strict)
SN Pull from Blocks 5-5-5-5-5
@80% of 1RM

WEEK 18 - FRI DEC 02 2011

PHASE I:
Games Track Athletes - Rest

WARMUP:
4 Rounds of
:15 Jumping Jack
:15 Squat
:15 MC
:15 Jump Squat

EQUIPMENT:
BB: 155/105

WOD:
7 Rounds of
PCL: 7
AbMat: 30

LIFTING/SKILL DEV:
Instructor Play

WEEK 18 - SAT DEC 03 2011

PHASE I:
Games Track Athletes - All

WARMUP:
4 Rounds of
:15 Jumping Jack
:15 Squat
:15 MC
:15 Jump Squat

EQUIPMENT: BB 135/95

WOD:
Amanda
MU
Snatch
9, 7, 5 for time

LIFTING/SKILL DEV:
No MU: Sub 3x Pull Ups/Dips
Then
Instructor Play

SKILL/DEV. WORK:
O-Lifting Class

GAMES WOD:
Death By Rope Climb

Week 19

	SUNDAY 12/4	MONDAY 12/5	TUESDAY 12/6
WARM UP	*Stove Pipe* **5 Rounds of** **A1** : Row 1:00 **A2** : Static KB Hold 1:00 *Transition :10*	Run/Lunge 2x Run/Bear Crawl 2x Run/Crab Walk: 2x Run/Inch Worm: 2x 30/20/30	*Tabata W/U* Squat Plank Hold Abmat Sit Up MC *16 intervals*
EQUIPMENT	Dynamax 20/14 BB 135/95	BB + Rack	BB
W O D	Wall Ball: 2-20 x 2 Pull Up: 1-10 x 1 PCL: 2-20 x 2 Burpee: 1-10 x 1	FSQ 3-3-3-3-3 *E3M* @90% of 1RM	DL 3-3-3-3-3 *E3M* @90% of 1RM
LIFTING/SKILL	*Instructor Play*	Ring Push Up *(from box)* Box Jump (24/20) Swing (24/16) *21, 15, 9 for time*	BSQ (95/65): 12 PJ: 10 *AMRAP: 4 Minutes -* *Rest 1:00 - 3 Rounds*
GAMES Phase I	Rest	All	All
SKILL/DEV WORK		Swing 10-10-10-10-10 *EMOTM #124/#88*	Swing 10-10-10-10-10 *EMOTM #124/#88*
GAMES WOD			
POWER HOUR All lifts E3M @90% of 1RM		FSQ 3-3-3-3-3 Push Jerk 3-3-3-3-3 SN 3-3-3-3-3	DL 3-3-3-3-3 Split Jerk 3-3-3-3-3

NOTES

132

WEDNESDAY 12/7	THURSDAY 12/8	FRIDAY 12/9	SATURDAY 12/10
Run/Lunge 2x Run/Bear Crawl 2x Run/Crab Walk 2x Run/Inch Worm 2x 30/20/30	Run/Lunge 2x Run/Bear Crawl 2x Run/Crab Walk: 2x Run/Inch Worm: 2x 30/20/30	Row 1k 30/20/30	**3 Rounds of** Jump Rope :45 - *Transition :15* Plank :45 - *Transition :15* Spidey L :45 - *Transition :15* Spidey R :45 - *Transition :15*
BB + Rack	BB + Rack	DB (2): #30/20	BB 155/105
OHS 3-3-3-3-3 @90% of 1RM	BSQ 3-3-3-3-3 *E3M* @90% of 1RM	Toes to Bar: 10 Rowing Push Up: 8 Thruster: 6 *AMRAP: 12 Minutes*	*DT* DL: 12 HPCL: 9 PJ: 6 *5 Rounds for time*
Wall Ball: 5 Burpee: 5 *AMRAP: 1 Minute - Rest* *1:00 - 10 Rounds*	PCL (135/95) Burpee *10, 9, 8, 7, 6, 5, 4, 3,* *2, 1 for time*	Row: 2k *Make sure you have* *time for two heats*	*Instructor Play*
All	**All**	**Rest**	**All**
Swing 10-10-10-10-10 *EMOTM #124/#88*	Swing 10-10-10-10-10 *EMOTM #124/#88*		
O-Lifting Class			*O-Lifting Class*
OHS 3-3-3-3-3 Pull Up (Strict)	BSQ 3-3-3-3-3 Press 3-3-3-3-3		

NOTES

WEEK 19 - SUN DEC 04 2011

PHASE I:
Games Track Athletes - Rest

WARMUP:
Stove Pipe:
P1: Row: 1:00
P2: Static KB Hold: 1:00
5 Rounds (:10 Transition)

EQUIPMENT:
Dynamax 20/14; BB 135/95

WOD:
Wall Ball: 2-20 x2
Pull Up: 1-10 x 1
PCL: 2-20 x 2
Burpee: 1-10 x 1

LIFTING/SKILL DEV:
Instructor Play

WEEK 19 - MON DEC 05 2011

PHASE I:
Games Track Athletes - All

WARMUP:
Run/Lunge 2x
Run/Bear Crawl 2x
Run/Crab Walk 2x
Run/Inch Worm 2x
30/20/30

EQUIPMENT: BB + Rack

WOD:
FSQ 3-3-3-3-3 E3M
@90% of 1RM

LIFTING/SKILL DEV:
Ring Push Up (from box)
Box Jump (24/20)
Swing (24/16)
21, 15, 9 for time

SKILL/DEV. WORK:
Swing 10-10-10-10-10
EMOTM (#124/#88)

POWER HOUR:
*NOTE: All strength sets
done every 3 minutes*
FSQ 3-3-3-3-3
@90% of 1RM
Push Jerk 3-3-3-3-3
@90% of 1RM
SN: 3-3-3-3-3
@90% of 1RM

WEEK 19 -
TUE DEC 06 2011

PHASE I:
Games Track Athletes - All

WARMUP:
Tabata W/U
Squat
Plank Hold
AbMat Sit Up
Mountain Climber
16 intervals

EQUIPMENT: BB

WOD:
DL 3-3-3-3-3 E3M
@90% of 1RM

LIFTING/SKILL DEV:
BSQ: 12 (95/65)
PJ: 10
AMRAP: 4 Minutes -
Rest 1:00 - 3 Rounds

SKILL/DEV. WORK:
Swing 10-10-10-10-10
EMOTM (#124/#88)

POWER HOUR:
*NOTE: All strength sets
done every 3 minutes*
DL 3-3-3-3-3
@90% of 1RM
Split Jerk 3-3-3-3-3
@90% of 1RM

WEEK 19 -
WED DEC 07 2011

PHASE I:
Games Track Athletes - All

WARMUP:
Run/Lunge 2x
Run/Bear Crawl 2x
Run/Crab Walk: 2x
Run/Inch Worm: 2x
30/20/30

EQUIPMENT: BB + Rack

WOD:
OHS 3-3-3-3-3 E3M
@90% of 1RM

LIFTING/SKILL DEV:
Wall Ball: 5
Burpee: 5
AMRAP: 1:00 - Rest 1:00 - 1
0 Rounds

SKILL/DEV. WORK:
NOTE: IN ADDITION TO WOD
Swing 10-10-10-10-10 EMOTM
(#124/#88)

GAMES WOD:
O-Lifting Class

POWER HOUR:
*NOTE: All strength sets
done every 3 minutes*
OHS 3-3-3-3-3 @90% of 1RM
Pull Up 3-3-3-3-3 (Strict)

WEEK 19 -
THU DEC 08 2011

PHASE I:
Games Track Athletes - All

WARMUP:
Run/Lunge 2x
Run/Bear Crawl 2x
Run/Crab Walk: 2x
Run/Inch Worm: 2x
30/20/30

EQUIPMENT: BB + Rack

WOD:
BSQ 3-3-3-3-3 E3M
@90% of 1RM

LIFTING/SKILL DEV:
PCL (135/95)
Burpee
10, 9, 8, 7, 6, 5, 4, 3, 2, 1
for time

SKILL/DEV. WORK:
Swing 10-10-10-10-10 EMOTM
(#124/#88)

POWER HOUR:
*NOTE: All strength sets
done every 3 minutes*
BSQ 3-3-3-3-3 @90% of 1RM
Press 3-3-3-3-3 @90% of 1RM

WEEK 19 -
FRI DEC 09 2011

PHASE I:
Games Track Athletes
- Rest

WARMUP:
Row 1k
30/20/30

EQUIPMENT:
DB (2): #30/20

WOD:
Toes to bar: 10
Rowing Push Up: 8
Thruster: 6
AMRAP: 12 Minutes

LIFTING/SKILL DEV:
Row: 2k for time -
Make sure you have
time for two heats

WEEK 19 -
SAT DEC 10 2011

PHASE I:
Games Track Athletes - All

WARMUP:
3 Rounds of
:45 Jump Rope
:15 Transition
:45 Plank
:15 Transition
:45 Spidey L
:15 Transition
:45 Spidey R
:15 Transition

EQUIPMENT:
BB 155/105

WOD:
DT
DL: 12
HPCL: 9
PJ: 6
5 Rounds for time

LIFTING/SKILL DEV:
Instructor Play

GAMES WOD:
O-Lifting Class

Week 20

	SUNDAY 12/11	MONDAY 12/12	TUESDAY 12/13
WARM UP	**4 Rounds of** :15 Jumping Jack :15 Squat :15 MC :15 Jump Squat	**4 Rounds of** :15 Jumping Jack :15 Squat :15 MC :15 Jump Squat	30/20/30 **Then 3 Rounds of** Burpee: 5 AbMat: 10
EQUIPMENT	C2 KB (2) 20kg/12kg KB 24kg/16kg	BB	BB + Rack
WOD	**A1** : Row 200 **A2** : KB Thrusters (Score) **A3** : Swing (Score) *AMRAP: 12* *Minutes*	DL 1-1-1-1-1-1-1 *E3M* Establish 1RM	OHS 1-1-1-1-1-1-1 *E3M* Establish 1RM
LIFTING/SKILL	*Instructor* *Games*	CL: 3 (185/120) Burpee: 9 *AMRAP: 12 Minutes*	CL&J *EMOTM for 15* *Minutes* HAP

GAMES Phase I	Rest	All	All
POWER HOUR **Max Effort** **Week** **All lifts** **Establish 1RM**		DL 1-1-1-1-1-1-1 Split Jerk 1-1-1-1-1-1-1 Clean from blocks 1-1-1-1-1-1	OHS 1-1-1-1-1-1-1 Pull Up (Strict) 1-1-1-1-1-1-1 Snatch from blocks 1-1-1-1-1-1-1

NOTES

138

WEDNESDAY 12/14	THURSDAY 12/15	FRIDAY 12/16	SATURDAY 12/17
30/20/30 **Then 3 Rounds of** Push Up: 5 AbMat: 10 Squat: 15	Row 500* 30/20/30 *If no rower, jump rope*	**4 Rounds of** :15 Jumping Jack :15 Squat :15 MC :15 Jump Squat	Jump Rope 5:00 30/20/30
BB + Rack	BB + Rack	BB 185/120 KB 24/16	Box 24/20 KB 16/12 BB 45/35
BSQ 1-1-1-1-1-1-1 *E3M* Establish 1RM	FSQ 1-1-1-1-1-1-1 *E3M* Establish 1RM	PCL: 3 Pull Up: 6 Swing: 9 *E2M for 30 Minutes (15 Rounds total)*	*Filthy 50:* Box jump: 50 Jumping pull-up: 50 Swing: 50 Lunge: 50 Knees to elbows: 50 Push press: 50 Back extension: 50 Wall ball: 50 Burpee: 50 Double under: 50
HPSN: 12 (95/65) Slam: 12 (20/14) Wall Ball: 12 *3 Rounds for time*	DL: 12 (225/145) Burpee: 10 *5 Rounds for time*		*Instructor Games*

All	All	Rest	All
BSQ 1-1-1-1-1-1-1 Press 1-1-1-1-1-1-1 CL&J 1-1-1-1-1-1-1	FSQ 1-1-1-1-1-1-1 Push Jerk 1-1-1-1-1-1-1		

NOTES

_____

_____

_____

WEEK 20 -
SUN DEC 11 2011

PHASE I:
Games Track Athletes - Rest

WARMUP:
4 Rounds of
:15 Jumping Jack
:15 Squat
:15 Mountain Climber
:15 Jump Squat

EQUIPMENT:
C2; KB (2) 20kg/12kg;
KB 24kg/16kg

WOD:
P1: Row: 200
P2: KB Thrusters (Score)
P3: Swing (Score)
AMRAP: 12 Minutes

LIFTING/SKILL DEV:
Instructor Games

WEEK 20 -
MON DEC 12 2011

PHASE I:
Games Track Athletes - All

WARMUP:
4 Rounds of
:15 Jumping Jack
:15 Squat
:15 Mountain Climber
:15 Jump Squat

EQUIPMENT: BB

WOD:
DL 1-1-1-1-1-1-1 E3M
Establish 1RM

LIFTING/SKILL DEV:
CL: 3 (185/120)
Burpee: 9
AMRAP: 12 Minutes

POWER HOUR:
DL 1-1-1-1-1-1-1
Establish 1RM
Split Jerk 1-1-1-1-1-1-1
Establish 1RM
Clean from block 1-1-1-1-1-1
Establish 1RM

WEEK 20 -
TUE DEC 13 2011

PHASE I:
Games Track Athletes - All

WARMUP:
30/20/30
Then 3 Rounds of
Burpee: 5
AbMat: 10

EQUIPMENT:
BB + Rack

WOD:
OHS 1-1-1-1-1-1-1 E3M
Establish 1RM

LIFTING/SKILL DEV:
CL&J EMOTM for 15 Minutes

POWER HOUR:
OHS 1-1-1-1-1-1-1
Establish 1RM
Pull Up 1-1-1-1-1-1-1
(Strict)
Snatch from block 1-1-1-1-1-1-1
Establish 1RM

WEEK 20 -
WED DEC 14 2011

PHASE I:
Games Track Athletes - All

WARMUP:
30/20/30
Then 3 Rounds of
Push Up: 5
AbMat: 10
Squat: 15

EQUIPMENT:
BB + Rack

WOD:
BSQ 1-1-1-1-1-1-1 E3M
Establish 1RM

LIFTING/SKILL DEV:
HPSN: 12 (95/65)
Slam: 12 (20/14)
Wall Ball: 12
3 Rounds for time

POWER HOUR:
BSQ 1-1-1-1-1-1-1
Establish 1RM
Press 1-1-1-1-1-1-1
Establish 1RM
CL&J 1-1-1-1-1-1-1
Establish 1RM

WEEK 20 - THU DEC 15 2011

PHASE I:
Games Track Athletes - All

WARMUP:
Row: 500*
30/20/30
*If no rower, jump rope

EQUIPMENT:
BB + Rack

WOD:
FSQ 1-1-1-1-1-1-1
E3M Establish 1RM

LIFTING/SKILL DEV:
DL: 12 (225/145)
Burpee: 10
5 Rounds for time

POWER HOUR:
FSQ 1-1-1-1-1-1-1
Establish 1RM
Push Jerk 1-1-1-1-1-1-1
Establish 1RM

WEEK 20 - FRI DEC 16 2011

PHASE I:
Games Track Athletes - Rest

WARMUP:
4 Rounds of
:15 Jumping Jack
:15 Squat
:15 Mountain Climber
:15 Jump Squat

EQUIPMENT:
BB 185/120; Kettlebell 24/16

WOD:
PCL: 3
Pull Up: 6
Swing: 9
E2M for 30 Minutes
(15 Rounds total)

WEEK 20 -
SAT DEC 17 2011

PHASE I:
Games Track Athletes - All

WARMUP:
Jump Rope: 5 Minutes
30/20/30

EQUIPMENT:
Box 24/20; KB 16/12;
BB 45/35

WOD:
Filthy 50
50 Box jump
50 Jumping pull-ups
50 Swings
50 Lunge
50 Knees to elbows
50 Push press
50 Back extensions
50 Wall ball
50 Burpees
50 Double unders

LIFTING/SKILL DEV:
Instructor Games

Week 21

	SUNDAY 12/18	MONDAY 12/19	TUESDAY 12/20
WARM UP	Row 1000 30/20/30	30/20/30 **Then BB Skills** DL/CL/FSQ/PP/BSQ *3 Reps each - 3 Rounds*	30/20/30 **Then 5 Rounds of** HPSN: 3 OHS: 3 HSN: 3
EQUIPMENT	BB 95/65	BB 95/65	BB + Weights
WOD	Row 1000 **Then** Thruster Pull Up *21, 15, 9 for* *time*	DL: 5 CL: 5 FSQ: 5 PP: 5 BSQ: 5 *AMRAP: 40 Minutes*	SN *EMOTM for 20* *Minutes*
LIFTING/SKILL			Slam: 12 (#30/#20) Wall Ball: 12 (#20/#14) *4 Rounds for time*
GAMES Phase I	Rest	All	All
SKILL/DEV WORK		5 Rounds of HSPU: 5 Dip: 5 DHPU: 5	5 Rounds of GHD H&B: 12 GHD Sit up: 12
GAMES WOD		MU: 3 BSQ: 10 (225/155) *7 Rounds for time*	DL: 30 (#135/95) Ring Dip: 10 *5 Rounds for time*
GAMES Accessory		*3 Rounds of* Reverse Hyper: 30 GHD Sit Up: 15	Cartwheel 40ft Hand Walk 40ft *5 Rounds (Play)*
POWER HOUR Conjugate Week		Butcher HiPush: 40ft #70/#50 Burpee: 10 *AMRAP: 15 Minutes*	Push Up: 6 Pull Up: 6 *EMOTM for 10 Minutes*

NOTES

_____

_____

_____

144

WEDNESDAY 12/21	THURSDAY 12/22	FRIDAY 12/23	SATURDAY 12/24
Run/Skip 2x Run/Lunge 2x Run/Bear Crawl 2x Run/Crab Walk 2x Run/Inch Worm 2x Run/Spidey 2x	**4 Rounds of** :15 Jumping Jack :15 Squat :15 MC :15 Jump Squat	Run/Skip 2x Run/Lunge 2x Run/Bear Crawl 2x Run/Crab Walk 2x Run/Inch Worm 2x Run/Spidey 2x	**4 Rounds of** :15 Jumping Jack :15 Squat :15 MC :15 Jump Squat
BB 95/65 KB 24/16kg	BB: 185/120		
Push Press: 21 Burpee: 15 American Swing: 9 *4 Rounds for time*	CL: 1 FSQ: 2 SJ: 1 *AMRAP: 15 Minutes*	Row 1000 **Then** Burpee: 15 Pull Up: 12 *4 Rounds for time*	***Fight Gone Bad***
DL: 1 Rep *every :15 for 20* *Rounds* (#315/205)	Push Up: Max Reps for :30 *Rest :30 - 10 Rounds* Total Reps)		
All	**All**	**Rest**	**All**
Rope Climb OHS (185/120) *5, 4, 3, 2, 1 (Completion)*	L-Sit - :30 Pistol: 10R/10L *5 Rounds (Completion)*		
Swing: 21 (40kg/24kg) T2B: 15 Thruster: 9 (135/95) *3 Rounds for time*	Swing: 50 (24/16) Wall Ball: 20 *5 Rounds for time*		
	HSPU: 3-3-3-3-3		
Rope Climb OHS (185/120) *5, 4, 3, 2, 1 (Completion)*	Butcher HiPush: 40ft #70/#50 Burpee: 10 *AMRAP: 15 Minutes*		

NOTES

_____

_____

_____

WEEK 21 -
SUN DEC 18 2011

PHASE I:
Games Track Athletes - Rest

WARMUP:
Row: 1000
30/20/30

EQUIPMENT:
BB 95/65

WOD:
Row: 1000
Then
Thruster
Pull Up
21, 15, 9 for time

WEEK 21 -
MON DEC 19 2011

PHASE I:
Games Track Athletes - All

WARMUP:
30/20/30
Then BB Skills
DL/CL/FSQ/PP/BSQ
3 Reps each - 3 rounds

EQUIPMENT: BB 95/65

WOD:
DL: 5
CL: 5
FSQ: 5
PP: 5
BSQ: 5
AMRAP: 40 Minutes

SKILL/DEV. WORK:
5 Rounds of
HSPU: 5
Dip: 5
DHPU: 5

GAMES WOD:
Muscle Up: 3
BSQ: 10 (#225/#155)
7 Rounds for time
ACCESSORY:
3 Rounds of
Reverse Hyper: 30
GHD Sit Up: 15

POWER HOUR:
NOTE: Conjugate Week
Butcher High Push: 40ft -
  #70/#50
Burpee: 10
AMRAP: 15 Minutes

WEEK 21 - TUE DEC 20 2011

PHASE I:
Games Track Athletes - All

WARMUP:
30/20/30
Then 5 Rounds of
HPSN: 3
OHS: 3
HSN: 3

EQUIPMENT: BB + Weights

WOD:
SN: EMOTM - 20 Minutes

LIFTING/SKILL DEV:
Slam: 12 (#30/#20)
Wall Ball: 12 (#20/#14)
4 Rounds for time

SKILL/DEV. WORK:
5 Rounds of
GHD H&B: 12
GHD Sit up: 12

GAMES WOD:
DL: 30 (#135/95)
Ring Dip: 10
5 Rounds for time

ACCESSORY:
Cartwheel 40ft
Hand Walk 40ft
5 Rounds (Play)

POWER HOUR:
NOTE: Conjugate Week
Push Up: 6
Pull Up: 6
EMOTM for 10 Minutes

WEEK 21 - WED DEC 21 2011

PHASE I:
Games Track Athletes - All

WARMUP:
Run/Skip 2x
Run/Lunge 2x
Run/Bear Crawl 2x
Run/Crab Walk 2x
Run/Inch Worm 2x
Run/Spidey 2x

EQUIPMENT:
BB 95/65; KB 24/16kg

WOD:
Push Press: 21
Burpee: 15
American Swing: 9
4 Rounds for time

LIFTING/SKILL DEV:
DL: 1 Rep every :15 for
20 Rounds (#315/205)

SKILL/DEV. WORK:
Rope Climb
OHS (185/120)
5, 4, 3, 2, 1 (Completion)

GAMES WOD:
Swing: 21 (40kg/24kg)
T2B: 15
Thruster: 9 (135/95)
3 Rounds for time

POWER HOUR:
NOTE: Conjugate Week
Rope Climb
OHS (185/120)
5, 4, 3, 2, 1 (Completion)

WEEK 21 - THU DEC 22 2011

PHASE I:
Games Track Athletes - All

WARMUP:
4 Rounds of
:15 Jumping Jack
:15 Squat
:15 Mountain Climber
:15 Jump Squat

EQUIPMENT: BB: 185/120

WOD:
CL: 1
FSQ: 2
SJ: 1
AMRAP: 15 Minutes

LIFTING/SKILL DEV:
Push Up: Max Reps for :30 -
Rest :30 - 10 Rounds
(Score Total Rep)

SKILL/DEV. WORK:
L-Sit :30
Pistol: 10R/10L
5 Rounds (Completion)

GAMES WOD:
Swing: 50 (24/16)
Wall Ball: 20
5 Rounds for time

ACCESSORY:
HSPU: 3-3-3-3-3

POWER HOUR:
NOTE: Conjugate Week
Butcher High Push:
40ft - #70/#50
Burpee: 10
AMRAP: 15 Minutes

WEEK 21 - FRI DEC 23 2011

PHASE I:
Games Track Athletes - Rest

WARMUP:
Run/Skip 2x
Run/Lunge 2x
Run/Bear Crawl 2x
Run/Crab Walk 2x
Run/Inch Worm 2x
Run/Spidey 2x

WOD:
Row: 1000
Then
Burpee: 15
Pull Up: 12
4 Rounds for time

WEEK 21 -
SAT DEC 24 2011

PHASE I:
Games Track Athletes - All

WARMUP:
4 Rounds of
:15 Jumping Jack
:15 Squat
:15 Mountain Climber
:15 Jump Squat

WOD:
Fight Gone Bad

NOTES

Week 22

	SUNDAY 12/25	MONDAY 12/26	TUESDAY 12/27
WARM UP	Wake Up Eat A Lot	**4 Rounds of** :15 Burpee :15 Swing :15 Squat :15 Lunge	**4 Rounds of** :15 Jumping Jack :15 Squats :15 Push Ups :15 Flutter Kicks
EQUIPMENT	Comatose on the couch	BB + Rack	BB + Rack
W O D	*Run: 10k*	BSQ: 5-5-5-5-5 *E3M* @80% of 1RM	FSQ: 5-5-5-5-5 *E3M* @80% of 1RM
LIFTING/SKILL	Stretch and Recover	PCL: 3 (185/120) Pull Up: 6 Swing: 9 (24/16) *AMRAP: 15 Minutes*	Burpee : 7 OHS: 7 (135/95) *7 Rounds for time*
GAMES Phase I	All	All	All
SKILL/DEV WORK		Rope Climb: 3 Double Under: 50 *3 Rounds - Completion*	OHS: 7 (185/120) Pull Up: 12 (#20 Vest) *3 Rounds - Completion*
GAMES W O D			
GAMES Accessory		Swing 10-10-10-10-10 #124/88	Swing 10-10-10-10-10 #124/88
POWER HOUR Week #1 All lifts @80% of 1RM		BSQ 5-5-5-5-5 Press 5-5-5-5-5 CL from Blocks 5-5-5-5-5	FSQ 5-5-5-5-5 Push Jerk 5-5-5-5-5 CL Pulls from Blocks 5-5-5-5-5

NOTES

150

WEDNESDAY 12/28	THURSDAY 12/29	FRIDAY 12/30	SATURDAY 12/31
4 Rounds of	**4 Rounds of**	**3 Rounds of**	*TBA*
:15 Burpee	:15 Jumping Jack	Row 2:00 - *Transition :15*	
:15 Swing	:15 Squats	Jump Rope 2:00 -	
:15 Squat	:15 Push Ups	*Transition :15*	
:15 Lunge	:15 Flutter Kicks		
BB + Rack	BB + Rack	KB - Heavy as possible	
DL: 5-5-5-5-5 *E3M*	OHS: 5-5-5-5-5 *E3M*	Turkish Get Up 1R/1L	*TBA*
@80% of 1RM	@80% of 1RM	*AMRAP: 10 Minutes*	
Thruster: 5 (95/65)	Low Box Jump: 15	DL: 15 (185/120)	
HPCL: 10	Cross Over Push Up: 10	Wall Ball: 15 (20/14)	
Ball Slam: 15 (30/20)	AbMat: 15	Ball Slam: 15 (30/20)	
5 Rounds for time	*AMRAP: 15 Minutes*	*5 Rounds for time*	
All	**All**	**Rest**	**All**
5 Rounds of	Wall Walk		*O-Lifting Class*
HSPU: 5	Cluster (185/120)		
GHD Sit Up: 15	*5, 4, 3, 2, 1*		
O-Lifting Class			
Swing 10-10-10-10-10	Swing 10-10-10-10-10		
#124/88	#124/88		
DL 5-5-5-5-5	OHS 5-5-5-5-5		
Split Jerk 5-5-5-5-5	Pull Up (Strict) 5-5-5-5-5		
SN from Blocks	SN Pull from Blocks		
5-5-5-5-5	5-5-5-5-5		

NOTES

_____

_____

_____

_____

WEEK 22 -
SUN DEC 25 2011

PHASE I:
Games Track Athletes - All

WARMUP:
Wake Up
Eat A Lot

EQUIPMENT:
Comatose on the couch

WOD:
Run: 10k

LIFTING/SKILL DEV:
Stretch and Recover

WEEK 22 -
MON DEC 26 2011

PHASE I:
Games Track Athletes - All

WARMUP:
4 Rounds of
:15 Burpee
:15 Swing
:15 Squat
:15 Lunge

EQUIPMENT: BB + Rack

WOD:
BSQ: 5-5-5-5-5 E3M
@80% of 1RM

LIFTING/SKILL DEV:
PCL: 3 (185/120)
Pull Up: 6
Swing: 9 (24/16)
AMRAP: 15 Minutes

SKILL/DEV. WORK:
Rope Climb: 3
Double Under: 50
3 Rounds - Completion

ACCESSORY:
Swing 10-10-10-10-10
(#124/#88)

POWER HOUR:
BSQ 5-5-5-5-5
@80% of 1RM
Press 5-5-5-5-5
@80% of 1RM
CL from Blocks 5-5-5-5-5
@80% of 1RM

152

WEEK 22 -
TUE DEC 27 2011

PHASE I:
Games Track Athletes - All

WARMUP:
4 Rounds of
:15 Jumping Jack
:15 Squats
:15 Push Ups
:15 Flutter Kicks

EQUIPMENT: BB + Rack

WOD:
FSQ: 5-5-5-5-5 E3M
@80% of 1RM

LIFTING/SKILL DEV:
Burpee : 7
OHS (135/95): 7
7 Rounds for time

SKILL/DEV. WORK:
OHS: 7 (185/120)
Pull Up: 12 (#20 Vest)
3 Rounds (Completion)

ACCESSORY:
Swing 10-10-10-10-10
(#124/#88)

POWER HOUR:
FSQ 5-5-5-5-5 @80% of 1RM
Push Jerk 5-5-5-5-5
@80% of 1RM
CL Pulls from Blocks 5-5-5-5-5
@80% of 1RM

WEEK 22 -
WED DEC 28 2011

PHASE I:
Games Track Athletes - All

WARMUP:
4 Rounds of
:15 Burpee
:15 Swing
:15 Squat
:15 Lunge

EQUIPMENT: BB + Rack

WOD:
DL: 5-5-5-5-5 E3M
@80% of 1RM

LIFTING/SKILL DEV:
Thruster: 5 (95/65)
HPCL: 10
Ball Slam: 15 (30/20)
5 Rounds for time

SKILL/DEV. WORK:
5 Rounds of
HSPU: 5
GHD Sit Up: 15

GAMES WOD:
O-Lifting Class

ACCESSORY:
Swing 10-10-10-10-10
(#124/#88)

POWER HOUR:
DL 5-5-5-5-5 @80% of 1RM
Split Jerk 5-5-5-5-5
@80% of 1RM
SN from Blocks 5-5-5-5-5
@80% of 1RM

**WEEK 22 -
THU DEC 29 2011**

PHASE I:
Games Track Athletes - All

WARMUP:
4 Rounds of
:15 Jumping Jack
:15 Squats
:15 Push Ups
:15 Flutter Kicks

EQUIPMENT: BB + Rack

WOD:
OHS: 5-5-5-5-5 E3M
@80% of 1RM

LIFTING/SKILL DEV:
Low Box Jump: 15
Cross Over Push Up: 10
AbMat: 15
AMRAP: 15 Minutes

SKILL/DEV. WORK:
Wall Walk
Cluster: (185/120)
5, 4, 3, 2, 1

ACCESSORY:
Swing 10-10-10-10-10
(#124/#88)

POWER HOUR:
OHS 5-5-5-5-5 @80% of 1RM
Pull Up 5-5-5-5-5 (Strict)
SN Pull from Blocks 5-5-5-5-5
@80% of 1RM

**WEEK 22 -
FRI DEC 30 2011**

PHASE I:
Games Track Athletes - Rest

WARMUP:
3 Rounds of
Row: 2:00 - :15 Transition
Jump Rope: 2:00 - :15 Transition

EQUIPMENT:
KB - Heavy as possible

WOD:
Turkish Get Up 1/1 -
AMRAP: 10 Minutes

LIFTING/SKILL DEV:
DL: 15 (185/120)
Wall Ball: 15 (20/14)
Ball Slam: 15 (30/20)
5 Rounds for time

WEEK 22 -
SAT DEC 31 2011

PHASE I:
Games Track Athletes - All

WARMUP:
TBA

WOD:
TBA

SKILL/DEV. WORK:
O-Lifting Class

Week 23

	SUNDAY 1/1	MONDAY 1/2	TUESDAY 1/3
WARM UP	**4 Rounds of** :15 Jumping Jack :15 Squat :15 MC :15 Jump Squat **Then 4 Rounds of** :15 Plank :15 Superman :15 Side Plank /R :15 Side Plank /L **Then** 30/20/30	**4 Rounds of** :15 Jumping Jack :15 Squat :15 MC :15 Jump Squat **Then 4 Rounds of** :15 Plank :15 Superman :15 Side Plank /R :15 Side Plank /L **Then** 30/20/30	**5 Rounds of** Jump Rope 1:00 Squat: 20 **Then 4 Rounds** :15 Plank :15 Superman :15 Side Plank /R :15 Side Plank /L
EQUIPMENT	BB #135/#95	BB + Rack	BB
W O D	BSQ: 20 Pull: 12 *AMRAP: 12* *Minutes*	FSQ: 3-3-3-3-3 *E3M* @90% of 1RM	DL: 3-3-3-3-3 *E3M* @90% of 1RM
LIFTING/SKILL		SDLHP: 12 (95/65) Push Jerk: 12 *5 Rounds for time*	Thruster: 3 Reps *every :30* *for 24 Intervals* (HAP)
GAMES Phase I	Rest	All	All
SKILL/DEV WORK		MU Transition: 10 DHPU: 10 Dip: 10 Ring Dips: 10 MU (Strict): 10 HSPU: 10 L-Sit - :20/:10 x 8 Rope Climbs: 5	TGU: 1R/1L x 10 Run: 400 x 6 - *Rest 1:00* Hand Walk: 40ft *Note: Sub wall walk: if no* *hand walk (15)*
GAMES W O D			Swing: 12-12-12-12-12 *EMOTM* #124/#88
GAMES Accessory			
POWER HOUR All lifts @90% of 1RM		PCL: 3-3-3-3-3	PSN: 3-3-3-3-3

156

WEDNESDAY 1/4	THURSDAY 1/5	FRIDAY 1/6	SATURDAY 1/7
Run/Lunge 2x Run/Bear Crawl 2x Run/Crab Walk 2x Run/Inch Worm 2x Run/Cart Wheel 2x 30/20/30	Run/Lunge 2x Run/Bear Crawl 2x Run/Crab Walk 2x Run/Inch Worm 2x Run/Cart Wheel 2x 30/20/30	Run/Lunge 2x Run/Bear Crawl 2x Run/Crab Walk 2x Run/Inch Worm 2x Run/Cart Wheel 2x **Then 4 Rounds of** :15 Jumping Jack :15 Squat :15 MC :15 Jump Squat **Then 4 Rounds of** :15 Plank :15 Superman :15 Side Plank /R :15 Side Plank /L **Then** 30/20/30	**4 Rounds of** :15 Jumping Jack :15 Squat :15 MC :15 Jump Squat **Then 4 Rounds of** :15 Plank :15 Superman :15 Side Plank /R :15 Side Plank /L *Then* 30/20/30
BB + Rack	BB + Rack	KB: 24/16kg DB: #35/#25	BB #135/#95
OHS 3-3-3-3-3 *E3M* @90% of 1RM	BSQ: 3-3-3-3-3 *E3M* @90% of 1RM	**A1** : Swing: 15 **A2** : Thruster (Score) **A3** : Box Jump (Score) *AMRAP: 15 Minutes*	DL: 9 HPSN: 6 OHS: 3 *5 Rounds for time*
Isabel: - (#135/#95) SN: 30 Reps *for time*	Push Up: 5 Pull Up: 5 *EMOTM for 20 Minutes*		
All	**All**	**Rest + Skill Work**	**All**
MU Transition: 10 DHPU: 10 Dip: 10 Ring Dips: 10 MU (Strict): 10 HSPU: 10 L-Sit - :20/:10 x 8 Rope Climbs: 5	TGU: 1R/1L x 10 Run: 400 x 6 - *Rest 1:00* Hand Walk: 40ft *Note: Sub wall walk: if no hand walk (15)*	Row: 5k (Recover & Stretch) Ankles up	
	Swing: 12-12-12-12-12 *EMOTM* #124/#88		Swing: 12-12-12-12-12 *EMOTM* #124/#88
Olympic Lifting			*Olympic Lifting*
CL: 3-3-3-3-3	SN: 3-3-3-3-3		

157

WEEK 23 -
SUN JAN 1 2012

PHASE I:
Games Track Athletes - Rest

WARMUP:
4 Rounds of
:15 Jumping Jack
:15 Squat
:15 Mountain Climber
:15 Jump Squat
Then 4 Rounds of
:15 Plank
:15 Superman
:15 Side Plank /R
:15 Side Plank /L
Then
30/20/30

EQUIPMENT: BB #135/#95

WOD:
BSQ: 20
Pull: 12
AMRAP: 12 Minutes

WEEK 23 -
MON JAN 02 2012

PHASE I:
Games Track Athletes - All

WARMUP:
4 Rounds of
:15 Jumping Jack
:15 Squat
:15 Mountain Climber
:15 Jump Squat
Then 4 Rounds of
:15 Plank
:15 Superman
:15 Side Plank /R
:15 Side Plank /L
Then
30/20/30

EQUIPMENT: BB + Rack

WOD:
FSQ: 3-3-3-3-3 E3M
@90% of 1RM

LIFTING/SKILL DEV:
SDLHP (95/65): 12
Push Jerk: 12
5 Rounds for time

SKILL/DEV. WORK:
MU Transitions: 10
DHPU: 10
Dip: 10
Ring Dips: 10
MU (Strict): 10
HSPU: 10
L-Sit - :20/:10 x 8
Rope Climbs: 5

POWER HOUR:
PCL: 3-3-3-3-3
@90% of 1RM

WEEK 23 -
TUE JAN 03 2012

PHASE I:
Games Track Athletes - All

WARMUP:
5 Rounds of
Jump Rope: 1:00
Squat: 20
Then 4 Rounds of
:15 Plank
:15 Superman
:15 Side Plank /R
:15 Side Plank /L

EQUIPMENT: BB

WOD:
DL: 3-3-3-3-3 E3M
@90% of 1RM

LIFTING/SKILL DEV:
Thruster: 3 Reps every -
:30 for 24 Intervals (HAP)

SKILL/DEV. WORK:
TGU: 1/1 x 10
Run: 400 x 6 - 1:00 Rest
Hand Walk: 40ft
Note: Sub wall walk:
if no hand walk (15)

GAMES WOD:
Swing: 12-12-12-12-12
EMOTM (#124/#88)

POWER HOUR:
PSN: 3-3-3-3-3 @90% of 1RM

WEEK 23 -
WED JAN 04 2012

PHASE I:
Games Track Athletes - All

WARMUP:
Run/Lunge 2x
Run/Bear Crawl 2x
Run/Crab Walk 2x
Run/Inch Worm 2x
Run/Cart Wheel 2x
30/20/30

EQUIPMENT: BB + Rack

WOD:
OHS 3-3-3-3-3 E3M
@90% of 1RM

LIFTING/SKILL DEV:
Isabel: - (#135/#95)
SN: 30 Reps for time

SKILL/DEV. WORK:
MU Transitions: 10
DHPU: 10
Dip: 10
Ring Dips: 10
MU (Strict): 10
HSPU: 10
L-Sit - :20/:10 x 8
Rope Climbs: 5

ACCESSORY:
Olympic Lifting

POWER HOUR:
CL: 3-3-3-3-3 @90% of 1RM

WEEK 23 -
THU JAN 05 2012

PHASE I:
Games Track Athletes - All

WARMUP:
Run/Lunge 2x
Run/Bear Crawl 2x
Run/Crab Walk 2x
Run/Inch Worm 2x
Run/Cart Wheel 2x
30/20/30

EQUIPMENT: BB + Rack

WOD:
BSQ: 3-3-3-3-3 E3M
@90% of 1RM

LIFTING/SKILL DEV:
Push Up: 5
Pull Up: 5
EMOTM for 20 Minutes

SKILL/DEV. WORK:
TGU: 1/1 x 10
Run: 400 x 6 - 1:00 Rest
Hand Walk: 40ft
Note: Sub wall walk:
if no hand walk (15)

GAMES WOD:
Swing: 12-12-12-12-12 EMOTM
(#124/#88)

POWER HOUR:
SN: 3-3-3-3-3 @90% of 1RM

WEEK 23 -
FRI JAN 06 2012

PHASE I:
Games Track Athletes -
Rest + Skill Work

WARMUP:
Run/Lunge 2x
Run/Bear Crawl 2x
Run/Crab Walk 2x
Run/Inch Worm 2x
Run/Cart Wheel 2x
Then 4 Rounds of
:15 Jumping Jack
:15 Squat
:15 Mountain Climber
:15 Jump Squat
Then 4 Rounds of
:15 Plank
:15 Superman
:15 Side Plank /R
:15 Side Plank /L
Then
30/20/30

EQUIPMENT:
KB: 24/16kg; DB: #35/#25

WOD:
P1: Swing: 15
P2: Thruster (Score)
P3: Box Jump (Score)

SKILL/DEV. WORK:
Row: 5k (Recover & Stretch)
Ankles up

WEEK 23 -
SAT JAN 07 2012

PHASE I:
Games Track Athletes - All

WARMUP:
4 Rounds of
:15 Jumping Jack
:15 Squat
:15 Mountain Climber
:15 Jump Squat
Then 4 Rounds of
:15 Plank
:15 Superman
:15 Side Plank /R
:15 Side Plank /L
Then
30/20/30

EQUIPMENT: BB #135/#95
WOD:
DL: 9
HPSN: 6
OHS: 3
5 Rounds for time

GAMES WOD:
Swing: 12-12-12-12-12 EMOTM
(#124/#88)

ACCESSORY:
Olympic Lifting

Week 24

	SUNDAY 1/8	MONDAY 1/9	TUESDAY 1/10
WARM UP	**4 Rounds of** :15 Jumping Jack :15 Squat :15 MC :15 Jump Squat **Then 4 Rounds of** :15 Plank :15 Superman :15 Side Plank /R :15 Side Plank /L **Then** 30/20/30	**4 Rounds of** :15 Jumping Jack :15 Squat :15 MC :15 Jump Squat **Then 4 Rounds of** :15 Plank :15 Superman :15 Side Plank /R :15 Side Plank /L **Then** 30/20/30	Row 1,000M 30/20/30
EQUIPMENT	KB: 24/16 DL: 185/120		
W O D	Swing: 30 Lunge: 20 Steps Deadlift: 10 *AMRAP: 20 Minutes*	DL: 1-1-1-1-1-1-1 *E3M* Establish 1RM	OHS: 1-1-1-1-1-1-1 *E3M* Establish 1RM
LIFTING/SKILL		*Karen*	*Cindy*
GAMES Phase I	Rest	All	All
SKILL/DEV WORK		MU Transition: 10 DHPU: 10 Dip: 10 Ring Dips: 10 MU (Strict): 10 HSPU: 10 L-Sit - :20/:10 x 8 Rope Climbs: 5	TGU: 1R/1L x 10 Run: 400 x 6 - *Rest 1:00* Hand Walk: 40ft *Note: Sub wall walk: if* *no hand walk (15)*
GAMES W O D			Swing: 12-12-12-12-12 *EMOTM* #124/#88
GAMES Accessory			
POWER HOUR All lifts Establish 1RM		PCL: 1-1-1-1-1-1-1	PSN: 1-1-1-1-1-1-1

162

WEDNESDAY 1/11	THURSDAY 1/12	FRIDAY 1/13	SATURDAY 1/14
4 Rounds of :15 Jumping Jack :15 Squat :15 MC :15 Jump Squat **Then 4 Rounds of** :15 Plank :15 Superman :15 Side Plank /R :15 Side Plank /L **Then** 30/20/30	Row 1,000M 30/20/30	**4 Rounds of** :15 Jumping Jack :15 Squat :15 MC :15 Jump Squat **Then 4 Rounds of** :15 Plank :15 Superman :15 Side Plank /R :15 Side Plank /L **Then** 30/20/30	Row 1,000M 30/20/30
			BB: 275/185 Box: 24/20
BSQ: 1-1-1-1-1-1-1 *E3M* Establish 1RM	FSQ: 1-1-1-1-1-1-1 *E3M* Establish 1RM	**A1** : Row 150 **A2** : Burpee (Score) **A3** : Thruster (Score) 35/25 *AMRAP: 12 Minutes*	DL: 5 Push Up: 13 Box Jump: 9 *AMRAP: 30 Minutes*
Fran	*Grace* *(PCL)*		
All	**All**	**Rest**	**All**
MU Transition: 10 DHPU: 10 Dip: 10 Ring Dips: 10 MU (Strict): 10 HSPU: 10 L-Sit - :20/:10 x 8 Rope Climbs: 5	TGU: 1R/1L x 10 Run: 400 x 6 - *Rest* *1:00* Hand Walk: 40ft *Note: Sub wall walk: if* *no hand walk (15)*	Row: 5k (Recover & Stretch) Ankles up	
	Swing: 12-12-12-12-12 *EMOTM* #124/#88		Swing: 12-12-12-12-12 *EMOTM* #124/#88
Olympic Lifting			*Olympic Lifting*
CL: 1-1-1-1-1-1-1	SN: 1-1-1-1-1-1-1		

163

WEEK 24 -
SUN JAN 08 2012

PHASE I:
Games Track Athletes - Rest

WARMUP:
4 Rounds of
:15 Jumping Jack
:15 Squat
:15 Mountain Climber
:15 Jump Squat
Then 4 Rounds of
:15 Plank
:15 Superman
:15 Side Plank /R
:15 Side Plank /L
Then
30/20/30

EQUIPMENT:
KB: 24/16; DL: 185/120

WOD:
Swing: 30
Lunge: 20 Steps
Deadlift: 10
AMRAP: 20 Minutes

WEEK 24 -
MON JAN 09 2012

PHASE I:
Games Track Athletes - All

WARMUP:
4 Rounds of
:15 Jumping Jack
:15 Squat
:15 Mountain Climber
:15 Jump Squat
Then 4 Rounds of
:15 Plank
:15 Superman
:15 Side Plank /R
:15 Side Plank /L
Then
30/20/30

WOD:
DL: 1-1-1-1-1-1-1 E3M
Establish 1RM

LIFTING/SKILL DEV:
Karen

SKILL/DEV. WORK:
MU Transitions: 10
DHPU: 10
Dip: 10
Ring Dips: 10
MU (Strict): 10
HSPU: 10
L-Sit - :20/:10 x 8
Rope Climbs: 5

POWER HOUR:
PCL: 1-1-1-1-1-1-1
Establish 1RM

WEEK 24 - TUE JAN 10 2012

PHASE I:
Games Track Athletes - All

WARMUP:
Row: 1,000M
30/20/30
WOD:
OHS: 1-1-1-1-1-1-1 E3M
Establish 1RM

LIFTING/SKILL DEV:
Cindy

SKILL/DEV. WORK:
TGU: 1/1 x 10
Run: 400 x 6 - 1:00 Rest
Hand Walk: 40ft
*Note: Sub wall walk:
if no hand walk (15)*

GAMES WOD:
Swing: 12-12-12-12-12
EMOTM (#124/#88)

POWER HOUR:
PSN: 1-1-1-1-1-1-1
Establish 1RM

WEEK 24 - WED JAN 11 2012

PHASE I:
Games Track Athletes - All

WARMUP:
4 Rounds of
:15 Jumping Jack
:15 Squat
:15 Mountain Climber
:15 Jump Squat
Then 4 Rounds of
:15 Plank
:15 Superman
:15 Side Plank /R
:15 Side Plank /L
Then
30/20/30

WOD:
BSQ: 1-1-1-1-1-1-1 E3M
Establish 1RM

LIFTING/SKILL DEV:
Fran

SKILL/DEV. WORK:
MU Transitions: 10
DHPU: 10
Dip: 10
Ring Dips: 10
MU (Strict): 10
HSPU: 10
L-Sit - :20/:10 x 8
Rope Climbs: 5

ACCESSORY:
Olympic Lifting

POWER HOUR:
CL: 1-1-1-1-1-1-1
Establish 1RM

165

**WEEK 24 -
THU JAN 12 2012**

PHASE I:
Games Track Athletes - All

WARMUP:
Row: 1,000M
30/20/30

WOD:
FSQ: 1-1-1-1-1-1-1 E3M
Establish 1RM

LIFTING/SKILL DEV:
Grace (PCL)

SKILL/DEV. WORK:
TGU: 1/1 x 10
Run: 400 x 6 - 1:00 Rest
Hand Walk: 40ft
Note: Sub wall walk:
if no hand walk (15)

GAMES WOD:
Swing: 12-12-12-12-12
EMOTM (#124/#88)

POWER HOUR:
SN: 1-1-1-1-1-1-1
Establish 1RM

**WEEK 24 -
FRI JAN 13 2011**

PHASE I:
Games Track Athletes - Rest

WARMUP:
4 Rounds of
:15 Jumping Jack
:15 Squat
:15 Mountain Climber
:15 Jump Squat
Then 4 Rounds of
:15 Plank
:15 Superman
:15 Side Plank /R
:15 Side Plank /L
Then
30/20/30

WOD:
P1: Row: 150
P2: Burpee (Score)
P3: Thruster 35/25 (Score)
AMRAP: 12 Minutes

SKILL/DEV. WORK:
Row: 5k (Recover & Stretch)
Ankles up

WEEK 24 -
SAT JAN 14 2011

PHASE I:
Games Track Athletes - All

WARMUP:
Row: 1,000M
30/20/30

EQUIPMENT:
BB: 275/185; Box: 24/20

WOD:
DL: 5
Push Up: 13
Box Jump: 9
AMRAP: 30 Minutes

GAMES WOD:
Swing: 12-12-12-12-12
EMOTM (#124/#88)

ACCESSORY:
Olympic Lifting

Week 25

	SUNDAY 1/15	MONDAY 1/16	TUESDAY 1/17
WARM UP	Low Box Jump: 10 Icky Shuffle Swing: 10 Icky Shuffle *AMRAP: 10 Minutes* **Then 4 Rounds of** :15 Jumping Jack :15 Squat :15 MC :15 Jump Squat **Then 4 Rounds of** :15 Plank :15 Superman :15 Side Plank /R :15 Side Plank /L	Low Box Jump: 10 Icky Shuffle Swing: 10 Icky Shuffle *AMRAP: 10 Minutes* **Then 4 Rounds of** :15 Jumping Jack :15 Squat :15 MC :15 Jump Squat **Then 4 Rounds of** :15 Plank :15 Superman :15 Side Plank /R :15 Side Plank /L	Lunge 40ft Push Up: 10 Lunge 40ft AbMat: 20 *AMRAP: 10 Minutes* **Then 4 Rounds of** :15 Jumping Jack :15 Squat :15 MC :15 Jump Squat **Then 4 Rounds of** :15 Plank :15 Superman :15 Side Plank /R :15 Side Plank /L
EQUIPMENT	Rings Dynamax (20/14)	Dumbbells 35/25 AbMat	Low Box BB 65/45
WOD	**A1** : Burpee: 10 **A2** : Ring Row (Score) **A3** : Wall Ball (Score) *AMRAP: 12 Minutes*	Alternating Thruster: 10 Pull Up: 10 AbMat: 10 *AMRAP: 20 Minutes*	**A1** : Row 250 **A2** : Low Box Jump (Score) **A3** : Push Press (Score) *AMRAP: 12 Minutes*
LIFTING/SKILL		Stretch and roll	
GAMES Phase I	Rest	All	All
SKILL/DEV WORK		MU Transition: 10 DHPU: 10 Dip: 10 Ring Dips: 10 MU (Strict): 10 HSPU: 10 L-Sit - :20/:10 x 8 Rope Climbs: 5	TGU: 1R/1L x 10 Run: 400 x 6 - *Rest 1:00* Hand Walk: 40ft *Note: Sub wall walk: if no hand walk (15)*
GAMES WOD		PCL&J (185/135) Double Under *5, 50, 4, 40, 3, 30, 2, 20, 1, 10 for time*	Swing: 12-12-12-12-12 *EMOTM #124/#88*
ACCESSORY			
POWER HOUR		SJ *EMOTM for 10 Minutes (HAP)*	DL/CL/FSQ/J - *AMRAP: 20 Minutes* (185/135)

168

WEDNESDAY 1/18	THURSDAY 1/19	FRIDAY 1/20	SATURDAY 1/21
Low Box Jump: 10	Lunge 40ft	**4 Rounds of**	**4 Rounds of**
Icky Shuffle	Push Up: 10	:15 Jumping Jack	:15 Jumping Jack
Swing: 10	Lunge 40ft	:15 Squat	:15 Squat
Icky Shuffle	AbMat: 20	:15 MC	:15 MC
AMRAP: 10 Minutes	*AMRAP: 10 Minutes*	:15 Jump Squat	:15 Jump Squat
Then 4 Rounds of	**Then 4 Rounds of**	**Then 4 Rounds of**	**Then 4 Rounds of**
:15 Jumping Jack	:15 Jumping Jack	:15 Plank	:15 Plank
:15 Squat	:15 Squat	:15 Superman	:15 Superman
:15 MC	:15 MC	:15 Side Plank /R	:15 Side Plank /R
:15 Jump Squat	:15 Jump Squat	:15 Side Plank /L	:15 Side Plank /L
Then 4 Rounds of	**Then 4 Rounds of**		
:15 Plank	:15 Plank		
:15 Superman	:15 Superman		
:15 Side Plank /R	:15 Side Plank /R		
:15 Side Plank /L	:15 Side Plank /L		
Box 24/20	Box 24/20		
KB 24/16	Rings		
Box Jump: 50	Box Jump: 10	*Two-Partner WOD*	*Diane*
Swing: 40	Ring Row: 10	Swing 2-20 x 2	
Burpee: 30	Ring Push Up: 10	Burpee 1-10 x 1	
Pull Up: 20	*AMRAP: 20 Minutes*	Thruster 2-20 x 2	
Dip: 10		Box Jump 1-10 x 1	
For time		Ball Slam 2-20 x 2	
		Games	
All	**All**	**Rest**	**All**
MU Transition: 10	TGU: 1R/1L x 10	Row: 5k (Recover &	
DHPU: 10	Run: 400 x 6 - *Rest 1:00*	Stretch)	
Dip: 10	Hand Walk: 40ft	Ankles up	
Ring Dips: 10	*Note: Sub wall walk: if no*		
MU (Strict): 10	*hand walk (15)*		
HSPU: 10			
L-Sit - :20/:10 x 8			
Rope Climbs: 5			
	Swing: 12-12-12-12-12		Swing: 12-12-12-12-12
	EMOTM #124/#88		*EMOTM #124/#88*
Olympic Lifting			***Olympic Lifting***
	HPSN: 5 (135/95)		
	Bench Press: 5 (185/135)		
	7 Rounds (completion)		

WEEK 25 - SUN JAN 15 2012

PHASE I:
Games Track Athletes - Rest

WARMUP:
Low Box Jump: 10
Icky Shuffle
Swing: 10
Icky Shuffle
AMRAP: 10 Minutes
Then 4 Rounds of
:15 Jumping Jack
:15 Squat
:15 Mountain Climber
:15 Jump Squat
Then 4 Rounds of
:15 Plank
:15 Superman
:15 Side Plank /R
:15 Side Plank /L

EQUIPMENT:
Rings; Dynamax (20/14)

WOD:
P1: Burpee: 10
P2: Ring Row (Score)
P3: Wall Ball (Score)

WEEK 25 - MON JAN 16 2012

PHASE I:
Games Track Athletes - All

WARMUP:
Low Box Jump: 10
Icky Shuffle
Swing: 10
Icky Shuffle
AMRAP: 10 Minutes
Then 4 Rounds of
:15 Jumping Jack
:15 Squat
:15 Mountain Climber
:15 Jump Squat
Then 4 Rounds of
:15 Plank
:15 Superman
:15 Side Plank /R
:15 Side Plank /L

EQUIPMENT:
Dumbbells 35/25; AbMat

WOD:
Alternating Thruster: 10
Pull Up: 10
AbMat: 10
AMRAP: 20 Minutes

LIFTING/SKILL DEV:
Stretch and roll

SKILL/DEV. WORK:
MU Transitions: 10
DHPU: 10
Dip: 10
Ring Dips: 10
MU (Strict): 10
HSPU: 10
L-Sit - :20/:10 x 8
Rope Climbs: 5

GAMES WOD:
PCL&J (185/135)
Double Under
5, 50, 4, 40, 3, 30, 2, 20, 1, 10
for time

POWER HOUR:
SJ: EMOTM for 10 Mins. (HAP)

WEEK 25 - TUE JAN 17 2012

PHASE I:
Games Track Athletes - All

WARMUP:
Lunge: 40ft
Push Up: 10
Lunge: 40ft
AbMat: 20
AMRAP: 10 Minutes
Then 4 Rounds of
:15 Jumping Jack
:15 Squat
:15 Mountain Climber
:15 Jump Squat
Then 4 Rounds of
:15 Plank
:15 Superman
:15 Side Plank /R
:15 Side Plank /L

EQUIPMENT:
Low Box; BB 65/45

WOD:
P1: Row 250
P2: Low Box Jump (Score)
P3: Push Press (Score)
AMRAP: 12 Minutes

SKILL/DEV. WORK:
TGU: 1/1 x 10
Run: 400 x 6 - 1:00 Rest
Hand Walk: 40ft
Note: Sub wall walk:
if no hand walk (15)

GAMES WOD:
Swing: 12-12-12-12-12
EMOTM (#124/#88)

POWER HOUR:
DL/CL/FSQ/J - AMRAP:
20 Minutes (185/135)

WEEK 25 - WED JAN 18 2012

PHASE I:
Games Track Athletes - All

WARMUP:
Low Box Jump: 10
Icky Shuffle
Swing: 10
Icky Shuffle
AMRAP: 10 Minutes
Then 4 Rounds of
:15 Jumping Jack
:15 Squat
:15 Mountain Climber
:15 Jump Squat
Then 4 Rounds of
:15 Plank
:15 Superman
:15 Side Plank /R
:15 Side Plank /L

EQUIPMENT:
Box 24/20; KB 24/16

WOD:
Box Jump: 50
Swing: 40
Burpee: 30
Pull Up: 20
Dip: 10
For time

SKILL/DEV. WORK:
MU Transitions: 10
DHPU: 10
Dip: 10
Ring Dips: 10
MU (Strict): 10
HSPU: 10
L-Sit - :20/:10 x 8
Rope Climbs: 5

ACCESSORY:
Olympic Lifting

WEEK 25 - THU JAN 19 2012

PHASE I:
Games Track Athletes - All

WARMUP:
Lunge: 40ft
Push Up: 10
Lunge: 40ft
AbMat: 20
AMRAP: 10 Minutes
Then 4 Rounds of
:15 Jumping Jack
:15 Squat
:15 Mountain Climber
:15 Jump Squat
Then 4 Rounds of
:15 Plank
:15 Superman
:15 Side Plank /R
:15 Side Plank /L

EQUIPMENT: Box 24/20; Rings

WOD:
Box Jump: 10
Ring Row: 10
Ring Push Up: 10
AMRAP: 20 Minutes

SKILL/DEV. WORK:
TGU: 1/1 x 10
Run: 400 x 6 - 1:00 Rest
Hand Walk: 40ft
Note: Sub wall walk:
if no hand walk (15)

GAMES WOD:
Swing: 12-12-12-12-12
EMOTM (#124/#88)

POWER HOUR:
HPSN: 5 (135/95)
Bench Press: 5 (185/135)
7 Rounds (for completion)

WEEK 25 - FRI JAN 20 2012

PHASE I:
Games Track Athletes - Rest

WARMUP:
4 Rounds of
:15 Jumping Jack
:15 Squat
:15 Mountain Climber
:15 Jump Squat
Then 4 Rounds of
:15 Plank
:15 Superman
:15 Side Plank /R
:15 Side Plank /L

WOD:
Two-Partner WOD
Swing 2-20 x 2
Burpee 1-10 x 1
Thruster 2-20 x 2
Box Jump 1-10 x 1
Ball Slam 2-20 x 2

LIFTING/SKILL DEV:
Games

SKILL/DEV. WORK:
Row: 5k (Recover & Stretch)
Ankles up

WEEK 25 -
SAT JAN 21 2102

PHASE I:
Games Track Athletes - All

WARMUP:
4 Rounds of
:15 Jumping Jack
:15 Squat
:15 Mountain Climber
:15 Jump Squat
Then 4 Rounds of
:15 Plank
:15 Superman
:15 Side Plank /R
:15 Side Plank /L

WOD:
Diane

GAMES WOD:
Swing: 12-12-12-12-12
EMOTM (#124/#88)

ACCESSORY:
Olympic Lifting

173

Week 26

	SUNDAY 1/22	MONDAY 1/23	TUESDAY 1/24
WARM UP	**4 Rounds of** :15 Jumping Jack :15 Squat :15 MC :15 Jump Squat **Then 4 Rounds of** :15 Plank :15 Superman :15 Side Plank /R :15 Side Plank /L	**4 Rounds of** :15 Jumping Jack :15 Squat :15 MC :15 Jump Squat **Then** Mobility ankles up - 5 Minutes	Run/Lunge 2x Run/Bear Crawl 2x Run/Crab Walk 2x Run/Inchworm 2x 30/20/30 Mobility ankles up - 5 Minutes
EQUIPMENT		BB + Rack	BB + Rack
WOD		BSQ: 5-5-5-5-5 *E3M* @80% of 1RM	FSQ: 5-5-5-5-5 *E3M* @80% of 1RM
LIFTING/SKILL	**A1** : Row: 200M **A2** : Double Under (Score) **A3** : Burpee (Score) *AMRAP: 12 Minutes*	Lunge (High Carry): 40ft (30/20) Push Press: 15 Lunge (High Carry): 40ft (30/20) Push Up: 15 *AMRAP: 20 Minutes*	
GAMES Phase 1	Rest	All	All
SKILL/DEV WORK		MU Transition: 10 DHPU: 10 Dip: 10 Double Unders: 100 Ring Dips: 10 MU (Strict): 10 HSPU: 10 L-Sit - :20/:10 x 8 Rope Climbs: 5	TGU: 1R/1L x 10 Run: 400 x 6 - *Rest 1:00* Hand Walk: 40ft *Note: Sub wall walk: if no hand walk (15)*
GAMES WOD		*Tabata Sprint - :20/:10 x 8* (ALL OUT)	Swing: 12-12-12-12-12 *EMOTM #124/#88* Slam: 10-10-10-10-10 *EMOTM #50/#40*
ACCESSORY			
POWER HOUR **All lifts** **@80% of RM**		PCL: 5-5-5-5-5 *EMOTM*	PSN: 5-5-5-5-5 *EMOTM*

WEDNESDAY 1/25	THURSDAY 1/26	FRIDAY 1/27	SATURDAY 1/28
4 Rounds of :15 Jumping Jack :15 Squat :15 MC :15 Jump Squat **Then** Mobility ankles up - 5 Minutes	30/20/30 **Then w/PVC Barbell** **Complex** *4 Rounds of* MSSN: 3 MSSN to OHS: 3 Dip to Catch: 3 Dip to Snatch:	**4 Rounds of** :15 Jumping Jack :15 Squat :15 MC :15 Jump Squat **Then** Mobility ankles up - 5 Minutes	**4 Rounds of** :15 Jumping Jack :15 Squat :15 MC :15 Jump Squat **Then** Mobility ankles up - 5 Minutes
BB	BB + Rack	Dynamax (20/14) KB: 24/16 Slammer #30/20	C2 BB 45/35
DL: 5-5-5-5-5 *E3M* @80% of 1RM	OHS: 5-5-5-5-5 *E3M* @80% of 1RM	A1 : Wall Ball 12 A2 : Swing (Score) A3 : Ball Slam: (Score) *AMRAP: 12 Minutes*	Row: 1000 Thruster: 50 Pull Up: 30 *For time*
Thruster (95/65) Burpee 5, 4, 3, 2, 1, 1, 2, 3, 4, 5 *For time*	Wall Ball: 50 (20/14) CL&J: 10 (135/95)	Row: 1k *for time*	*Instructor Play*
All	**All**	**Rest**	**All**
MU Transition: 10 DHPU: 10 Dip: 10 Double Unders: 100 Ring Dips: 10 MU (Strict): 10 HSPU: 10 L-Sit - :20/:10 x 8 Rope Climbs: 5	TGU: 1R/1L x 10 Run: 400 x 6 - *Rest 1:00* Hand Walk: 40ft *Note: Sub wall walk: if* *no hand walk (15)*	Do WARMUP for class Row: 5k (Recovery & Stretch)	
Tabata Sprint - :20/:10 *x 8 (ALL OUT)*	Swing: 12-12-12-12-12 *EMOTM #124/#88* Slam: 10-10-10-10-10 *EMOTM #50/#40*		Swing: 12-12-12-12-12 *EMOTM #124/#88*
Olympic Lifting			*Olympic Lifting*
CL: 5-5-5-5-5 *EMOTM*	SN: 5-5-5-5-5 *EMOTM*		

WEEK 26 - SUN JAN 22 2012

PHASE I:
Games Track Athletes - Rest

WARMUP:
4 Rounds of
:15 Jumping Jack
:15 Squat
:15 Mountain Climber
:15 Jump Squat
Then 4 Rounds of
:15 Plank
:15 Superman
:15 Side Plank /R
:15 Side Plank /L

LIFTING/SKILL DEV:
P1: Row: 200M
P2: Double Under (Score)
P3: Burpee (Score)
AMRAP: 12 Minutes

WEEK 26 - MON JAN 23 2012

PHASE I:
Games Track Athletes - All

WARMUP:
4 Rounds of
:15 Jumping Jack
:15 Squat
:15 Mountain Climber
:15 Jump Squat
Then
Mobility ankles up - 5 Minutes

EQUIPMENT: BB + Rack

WOD:
BSQ: 5-5-5-5-5 E3M
@80% of 1RM

LIFTING/SKILL DEV:
Lunge (High Carry):
40ft - 30/20
Push Press: 15
Lunge (High Carry):
40ft - 30/20
Push Up: 15
AMRAP: 20 Minutes

SKILL/DEV. WORK:
MU Transitions: 10
DHPU: 10
Dip: 10
Double Unders: 100
Ring Dips: 10
MU (Strict): 10
HSPU: 10
L-Sit - :20/:10 x 8
Rope Climbs: 5

GAMES WOD:
Tabata Sprint :20/:10 x 8
(ALL OUT)

POWER HOUR:
PCL: 5-5-5-5-5 EMOTM
@80% of 1RM

WEEK 26 -
TUE JAN 24 2012

PHASE I:
Games Track Athletes - All

WARMUP:
Run/Lunge 2x
Run/Bear Crawl 2x
Run/Crab Walk 2x
Run/Inchworm 2x
30/20/30
Mobility ankles up - 5 Minutes

EQUIPMENT: BB + Rack

WOD:
FSQ: 5-5-5-5-5 E3M
@80% of 1RM

LIFTING/SKILL DEV:
Thruster (95/65)
Burpee
5, 4, 3, 2, 1, 1, 2, 3, 4, 5
For time

SKILL/DEV. WORK:
TGU: 1/1 x 10
Run: 400 x 6 - 1:00 Rest
Hand Walk: 40ft
Note: Sub wall walk:
if no hand walk (15)

GAMES WOD:
Swing: 12-12-12-12-12
EMOTM (#124/#88)
Slam: 10-10-10-10-10
EMOTM (#50/#40)

POWER HOUR:
PSN: 5-5-5-5-5 EMOTM
@80% of 1RM

WEEK 26 -
WED JAN 25 2012

PHASE I:
Games Track Athletes - All

WARMUP:
4 Rounds of
:15 Jumping Jack
:15 Squat
:15 Mountain Climber
:15 Jump Squat
Then
Mobility ankles up - 5 Minutes

EQUIPMENT: BB

WOD:
DL: 5-5-5-5-5 E3M
@80% of 1RM

LIFTING/SKILL DEV:
Wall Ball: 50 (20/14)
CL&J: 10 (135/95)

SKILL/DEV. WORK:
MU Transitions: 10
DHPU: 10
Dip: 10
Double Unders: 100
Ring Dips: 10
MU (Strict): 10
HSPU: 10
L-Sit - :20/:10 x 8
Rope Climbs: 5

GAMES WOD:
Tabata Sprint :20/:10 x 8
(ALL OUT) -
On Woodway Curve

ACCESSORY:
Olympic Lifting

POWER HOUR:
CL: 5-5-5-5-5 EMOTM
@80% of 1RM

WEEK 26 -
THU JAN 26 2012

PHASE I:
Games Track Athletes - All

WARMUP:
30/20/30
Then w/PVC
4 Rounds of
MSSN: 3
MSSN to OHS: 3
Dip to Catch: 3
Dip to Snatch: 3

EQUIPMENT: BB + Rack

WOD:
OHS: 5-5-5-5-5 E3M
@80% of 1RM

LIFTING/SKILL DEV:
Row: 1k for time

SKILL/DEV. WORK:
TGU: 1/1 x 10
Run: 400 x 6 - 1:00 Rest
Hand Walk: 40ft
Note: Sub wall walk:
if no hand walk (15)

GAMES WOD:
Swing: 12-12-12-12-12
EMOTM (#124/#88)
Slam: 10-10-10-10-10
EMOTM (#50/#40)

POWER HOUR:
SN: 5-5-5-5-5 EMOTM
@80% of 1RM

WEEK 26 -
FRI JAN 27 2012

PHASE I:
Games Track Athletes - Rest

WARMUP:
4 Rounds of
:15 Jumping Jack
:15 Squat
:15 Mountain Climber
:15 Jump Squat
Then
Mobility ankles up - 5 Minutes

EQUIPMENT:
Dynamax (20/14); KB: 24/16;
Slammer #30/20

WOD:
P1: Wall Ball 12
P2: Swing (Score)
P3: Ball Slam: (Score)
AMRAP: 12 Minutes

LIFTING/SKILL DEV:
Instructor Play

SKILL/DEV. WORK:
Do WARMUP for class
Row: 5k (Recover & Stretch)

WEEK 26 -
SAT JAN 28 2012

PHASE I:
Games Track Athletes - All

WARMUP:
4 Rounds of
:15 Jumping Jack
:15 Squat
:15 Mountain Climber
:15 Jump Squat
Then
Mobility ankles up - 5 Minutes

EQUIPMENT:
C2; BB 45/35

WOD:
Row: 1000
Thruster: 50
Pull Up: 30
For time

GAMES WOD:
Swing: 12-12-12-12-12
EMOTM (#124/#88)

ACCESSORY:
Olympic Lifting

Week 27

	SUNDAY 1/29	MONDAY 1/30	TUESDAY 1/31
WARM UP	A-skip/run: 3 B-skip/run: 3 C-skip/run: 3 Run/Lunge 3x Run/Bear Crawl 3x Run/Crab Walk 3x Run/Inch Worm 3x Run/Spidey 3x	:15 Jumping Jack :15 Air Squat :15 MC :15 Jump Squat *4 Rounds for time*	:15 Jumping Jack :15 Air Squat :15 MC :15 Jump Squat *4 Rounds for time*
EQUIPMENT	AbMat		
WOD	*Partners WOD* Squat 5-25 x 5 Push Up: 1-10 x 1 AbMat: 5-25 x 5 Burpee: 1-10 x 1	FSQ: 3-3-3-3-3 *E3M* @90% of 1RM	DL: 3-3-3-3-3 *E3M* @90% of 1RM
LIFTING/SKILL		Press: 3 (#95/#65) Push Press: 6 Push Jerk: 9 SDLHP: 12 *3 Rounds for time*	Swing: 50 (24kg/16kg) Burpee: 20 *3 Rounds for time*
GAMES Phase I	Rest	All	All
SKILL/DEV WORK		MU Transition: 10 DHPU: 10 Dip: 10 Ring Dips: 10 MU (Strict): 10 HSPU: 10 L-Sit - :20/:10 x 8 Rope Climbs: 5	TGU: 1R/1L x 10 Run: 400 x 6 - *Rest 1:00* Hand Walk: 40ft *Note: Sub wall walk: if no hand walk (15)*
GAMES WOD		Sprint :30 - *Rest :30* - *10 Rounds*	Swing: 12-12-12-12-12 *EMOTM #124/#88*
ACCESSORY			
POWER HOUR All lifts @90% of RM		PCL: 3-3-3-3-3 From Blocks	PSN: 3-3-3-3-3 From Blocks

WEDNESDAY 2/1	THURSDAY 2/2	FRIDAY 2/3	SATURDAY 2/4
:15 Jumping Jack :15 Air Squat :15 MC :15 Jump Squat *4 Rounds for time*	:15 Jumping Jack :15 Air Squat :15 MC :15 Jump Squat *4 Rounds for time*	:15 Jumping Jack :15 Air Squat :15 MC :15 Jump Squat *4 Rounds for time*	:15 Jumping Jack :15 Air Squat :15 MC :15 Jump Squat *4 Rounds for time*
		KB: 32/24	
OHS: 3-3-3-3-3 *E3M* @90% of 1RM	BSQ: 3-3-3-3-3 *E3M* @90% of 1RM	Row 1000 *Then* American Swing Clean and Jerk *15, 12, 9 for time*	*Roy*
Wall Ball: 10 (20/14) *EMOTM for 10 Minutes*	Row: 500 Air Squat: 40 Sit Up: 30 Push Up: 20 Pull Up: 10 *For time*	*Fun and games*	
All	**All**	**Rest**	**All**
MU Transition: 10 DHPU: 10 Dip: 10 Ring Dips: 10 MU (Strict): 10 HSPU: 10 L-Sit - :20/:10 x 8 Rope Climbs: 5	TGU: 1R/1L x 10 Run: 400 x 6 - *Rest 1:00* Hand Walk: 40ft *Note: Sub wall walk: if no* *hand walk (15)*	Row: 5k (Recover & Stretch) Ankles up	*Winter Challenge*
Sprint :30 - *Rest :30* *- 10 Rounds*	Swing: 12-12-12-12-12 *EMOTM #124/#88*		
Olympic Lifting			
CL: 3-3-3-3-3 From Blocks	SN: 3-3-3-3-3 From Blocks		

WEEK 27 -
SUN JAN 29 2012

PHASE I:
Games Track Athletes - Rest

WARMUP:
A-skip/run: 3
B-skip/run: 3
C-skip/run:3
Run/Lunge 3x
Run/Bear Crawl 3x
Run/Crab Walk 3x
Run/Inch Worm 3x
Run/Spidey 3x

EQUIPMENT:
AbMat

WOD:
Partners
Squat 5-25 x 5
Push Up: 1-10 x 1
AbMat: 5-25 x 5
Burpee: 1-10 x 1

WEEK 27 -
MON JAN 30 2012

PHASE I:
Games Track Athletes - All

WARMUP:
:15 Jumping Jack
:15 Air Squat
:15 Mountain Climber
:15 Jump Squat
4 Rounds for time

WOD:
FSQ: 3-3-3-3-3 E3M
@90% of 1RM

LIFTING/SKILL DEV:
Press: 3 (#95/#65)
Push Press: 6
Push Jerk: 9
SDLHP: 12
3 Rounds for time

SKILL/DEV. WORK:
MU Transitions: 10
DHPU: 10
Dip: 10
Ring Dips: 10
MU (Strict): 10
HSPU: 10
L-Sit - :20/:10 x 8
Rope Climbs: 5

GAMES WOD:
Sprint :30 - :30 Rest -
10 Rounds

POWER HOUR:
PCL from Blocks:
3-3-3-3-3 @90% of 1RM

WEEK 27 -
TUE JAN 31 2012

PHASE I:
Games Track Athletes - All

WARMUP:
:15 Jumping Jack
:15 Air Squat
:15 Mountain Climber
:15 Jump Squat
4 Rounds for time

WOD:
DL: 3-3-3-3-3 E3M
@90% of 1RM

LIFTING/SKILL DEV:
Swing: 50 (24kg/16kg)
Burpee: 20
3 Rounds for time

SKILL/DEV. WORK:
TGU: 1/1 x 10
Run: 400 x 6 - 1:00 Rest
Hand Walk: 40ft
Note: Sub wall walk:
if no hand walk (15)

GAMES WOD:
Swing: 12-12-12-12-12
EMOTM (#124/#88)

POWER HOUR:
PSN from Blocks: 3-3-3-3-3
@90% of 1RM

WEEK 27 -
WED FEB 01 2012

PHASE I:
Games Track Athletes - All

WARMUP:
:15 Jumping Jack
:15 Air Squat
:15 Mountain Climber
:15 Jump Squat
4 Rounds for time

WOD:
OHS: 3-3-3-3-3 E3M
@90% of 1RM

LIFTING/SKILL DEV:
Wall Ball: 10 EMOTM for
10 Minutes (20/14)

SKILL/DEV. WORK:
MU Transitions: 10
DHPU: 10
Dip: 10
Ring Dips: 10
MU (Strict): 10
HSPU: 10
L-Sit - :20/:10 x 8
Rope Climbs: 5

GAMES WOD:
Sprint :30 - :30 Rest -
10 Rounds

ACCESSORY:
Olympic Lifting

POWER HOUR:
CL from Blocks: 3-3-3-3-3
@90% of 1RM

WEEK 27 - THU FEB 02 2012

PHASE I:
Games Track Athletes - All

WARMUP:
:15 Jumping Jack
:15 Air Squat
:15 Mountain Climber
:15 Jump Squat
4 Rounds for time

WOD:
BSQ: 3-3-3-3-3 E3M
@90% of 1RM

LIFTING/SKILL DEV:
Row: 500
Air Squat: 40
Sit Up: 30
Push Up: 20
Pull Up: 10
For time

SKILL/DEV. WORK:
TGU: 1/1 x 10
Run: 400 x 6 - 1:00 Rest
Hand Walk: 40ft
*Note: Sub wall walk:
if no hand walk (15)*

GAMES WOD:
Swing: 12-12-12-12-12 EMOTM
(#124/#88)

POWER HOUR:
SN from Blocks: 3-3-3-3-3
@90% of 1RM

WEEK 27 - FRI FEB 03 2012

PHASE I:
Games Track Athletes - Rest

WARMUP:
:15 Jumping Jack
:15 Air Squat
:15 Mountain Climber
:15 Jump Squat
4 Rounds for time

EQUIPMENT: KB: 32/24

WOD:
Row: 1000
Then
American Swing
Clean and Jerk
15, 12, 9 for time

LIFTING/SKILL DEV:
Fun and games

SKILL/DEV. WORK:
Row: 5k (Recover & Stretch)
Ankles up

184

**WEEK 27 -
SAT FEB 04 2012**

PHASE I:
Games Track Athletes - All

WARMUP:
:15 Jumping Jack
:15 Air Squat
:15 Mountain Climber
:15 Jump Squat
4 Rounds for time

WOD:
Roy

SKILL/DEV. WORK:
Winter Challenge

Week 28

	SUNDAY 2/5	MONDAY 2/6	TUESDAY 2/7
WARM UP	**4 Rounds of** :15 Jumping Jack :15 Squat :15 MC :15 Jump Squat **Then** 30/20/30	**4 Rounds of** :15 Jumping Jack :15 Squat :15 MC :15 Jump Squat **Then** 30/20/30	**4 Rounds of** :15 Jumping Jack :15 Squat :15 MC :15 Jump Squat **Then** 30/20/30
EQUIPMENT	BB 275/185 BB 95/65	BB + Weights	BB + Weights
W O D	*Quarter Gone Bad* *Format: Work :15 -* *Rest :45* Deadlift Thruster Pull Up Burpee *5 Rounds for Reps*	DL: 1-1-1-1-1-1-1 *E3M* Establish 1RM	OHS: 1-1-1-1-1-1-1 *E3M* Establish 1RM
LIFTING/SKILL		Push Jerk: 20 (135/95) Air Squat: 100 *2 Rounds for time*	OHS (#95/#65) Ring Push Up Ring Row *21, 15, 9 for time*
GAMES Phase I	Rest	All	All
SKILL/DEV WORK	MU Transition: 10 DHPU: 10 Dip: 10 Ring Dips: 10 MU (Strict): 10 HSPU: 10 L-Sit - :20/:10 x 8 Rope Climbs: 5	TGU: 1R/1L x 10 Run: 400 x 6 -*Rest 1:00* Hand Walk 40ft *Note: Sub wall walk: if* *no hand walk (15)*	MU Transition: 10 DHPU: 10 Dip: 10 Ring Dips: 10 MU (Strict): 10 HSPU: 10 L-Sit - :20/:10 x 8 Rope Climbs: 5
GAMES W O D		10 Rope Climbs *for time*	Swing: 12-12-12-12-12 *EMOTM* #124/#88
ACCESSORY		Ring Support - :20/:10 x 8 Ring Dip Bottom - :20/:10 x 8	GHD Sit Up: 15 GHD H & B Ext: 15 *3 Rounds (completion)*
POWER HOUR All lifts @90% of RM		PCL from Blocks: 3-3-3-3-3	PSN from Blocks: 3-3-3-3-3

WEDNESDAY 2/8	THURSDAY 2/9	FRIDAY 2/10	SATURDAY 2/11
4 Rounds of :15 Jumping Jack :15 Squat :15 MC :15 Jump Squat **Then** 30/20/30	**4 Rounds of** :15 Jumping Jack :15 Squat :15 MC :15 Jump Squat **Then** 30/20/30	**4 Rounds of** :15 Jumping Jack :15 Squat :15 MC :15 Jump Squat **Then** 30/20/30	**4 Rounds of** :15 Jumping Jack :15 Squat :15 MC :15 Jump Squat **Then** 30/20/30
BB + Weights	BB + Weights	Handles or KBs	BB: 225/155 Box: 24/20
BSQ: 1-1-1-1-1-1-1 *E3M* Establish 1RM	FSQ: 1-1-1-1-1-1-1 *E3M* Establish 1RM	**A1** : Farmer's Carry: 100ft (90/70) **A2** : AbMat Sit Up (Score) **A3** : Burpee *AMRAP: 10 Minutes*	*Roy:* DL: 15 Box Jump: 20 Pull Up: 25 *5 Rounds for time*
5 Rounds of Thruster: 7 (#95/#65) Ball Slam: 12 (#30/#20)	Row: 1000M *Then* SDLHP: 11 (#95/#65) PJ: 7 *3 Rounds for time*	***Rope Climb Skills***	
All	**All**	**Only Skill/Dev Work**	**All**
TGU: 1R/1L x 10 Run: 400 x 6 - *Rest* *1:00* Hand Walk: 40ft *Note: Sub wall walk: if* *no hand walk (15)*	Row: 5k (Recover & Stretch) Ankles up		
Butcher HiPush: 40ft (#70/#50) Burpee: 10 *AMRAP: 10 Minutes*	Swing: 12-12-12-12-12 *EMOTM #124/#88*		Swing: 12-12-12-12-12 *EMOTM #124/#88*
Olympic Lifting	GHD Sit Up: 15 GHD H & B Ext: 15 *3 Rounds (completion)*		***Olympic Lifting***
CL from Blocks: 3-3-3-3-3	SN from Blocks: 3-3-3-3-3		

WEEK 28 - SUN FEB 05 2012

PHASE I:
Games Track Athletes - Rest

WARMUP:
4 Rounds of
:15 Jumping Jack
:15 Squat
:15 Mountain Climber
:15 Jump Squat
Then
30/20/30

EQUIPMENT:
BB #275/#185; BB #95/#65

WOD:
Quarter Gone Bad
Format: Work for :15
- Rest for :45
Deadlift
Thruster
Pull Up
Burpee
5 Rounds for Reps

WEEK 28 - MON FEB 06 2012

PHASE I:
Games Track Athletes - All

WARMUP:
4 Rounds of
:15 Jumping Jack
:15 Squat
:15 Mountain Climber
:15 Jump Squat
Then
30/20/30

EQUIPMENT: BB + Weights

WOD:
DL 1-1-1-1-1-1-1 E3M
Establish 1RM

LIFTING/SKILL DEV:
Push Jerk: 20 (#135/#95)
Air Squat: 100
2 Rounds for time

SKILL/DEV. WORK:
MU Transitions: 10
DHPU: 10
Dips: 10
Ring Dip: 10
MU: 10 (Strict)
HSPU: 10
L-Sit - :20/:10 x 8
Rope Climb: 5

GAMES WOD:
10 Rope Climbs for time

ACCESSORY:
Ring Support - :20/:10 x 8
Ring Dip Bottom - :20/:10 x 8

POWER HOUR:
PCL from Blocks 3-3-3-3-3

WEEK 28 -
TUE FEB 07 2012

PHASE I:
Games Track Athletes - All

WARMUP:
4 Rounds of
:15 Jumping Jack
:15 Squat
:15 Mountain Climber
:15 Jump Squat
Then
30/20/30

EQUIPMENT: BB + Weights

WOD:
OHS 1-1-1-1-1-1-1 E3M
Establish 1RM

LIFTING/SKILL DEV:
OHS: (#95/#65)
Ring Push Up
Ring Row
21, 15, 9 for time

SKILL/DEV. WORK:
TGU: 1/1 x 10
Run: 400 x 6 - 1:00 Rest
Hand Walk 40ft
*Note: Sub wall walk
if no hand walk (15)*

GAMES WOD:
Swing: 12-12-12-12-12 EMOTM
(#124/#88)

ACCESSORY:
GHD Sit Up: 15
GHD H & B Ext: 15
3 Rounds for completion

POWER HOUR:
PSN from Blocks 3-3-3-3-3

WEEK 28 -
WED FEB 08 2012

PHASE I:
Games Track Athletes - All

WARMUP:
4 Rounds of
:15 Jumping Jack
:15 Squat
:15 Mountain Climber
:15 Jump Squat
Then 30/20/30

EQUIPMENT: BB + Weights

WOD:
BSQ 1-1-1-1-1-1-1 E3M
Establish 1RM

LIFTING/SKILL DEV:
5 Rounds of
Thruster: 7 (#95/#65)
Ball Slam: 12 (#30/#20)

SKILL/DEV. WORK:
MU Transitions: 10
DHPU: 10
Dips: 10
Ring Dip: 10
MU: 10 (Strict)
HSPU: 10
L-Sit - :20/:10 x 8
Rope Climb: 5

GAMES WOD:
Butcher High Push: 40ft
(#70/#50)
Burpee: 10
AMRAP: 10 Minutes

ACCESSORY:
Olympic Lifting

POWER HOUR:
CL from Blocks 3-3-3-3-3

189

WEEK 28 -
THU FEB 09 2012

PHASE I:
Games Track Athletes - All

WARMUP:
4 Rounds of
:15 Jumping Jack
:15 Squat
:15 Mountain Climber
:15 Jump Squat
Then 30/20/30

EQUIPMENT: BB + Weights

WOD:
FSQ 1-1-1-1-1-1-1 E3M
Establish 1RM

LIFTING/SKILL DEV:
Row: 1000M
Then
SDLHP: 11 (#95/#65)
PJ: 7
3 Rounds for time

SKILL/DEV. WORK:
TGU: 1/1 x 10
Run: 400 x 6 - 1:00 Rest
Hand Walk: 40ft
Note: Sub wall walk
if no hand walk (15)

GAMES WOD:
Swing: 12-12-12-12-12
EMOTM (#124/#88)

ACCESSORY:
GHD Sit Up: 15
GHD H & B Ext: 15
3 Rounds for completion

POWER HOUR:
SN from Blocks 3-3-3-3-3

WEEK 28 -
FRI FEB 10 2012

PHASE I:
Games Track Athletes -
Active Rest

WARMUP:
4 Rounds of
:15 Jumping Jack
:15 Squat
:15 Mountain Climber
:15 Jump Squat
Then
30/20/30

EQUIPMENT:
Handles or KBs

WOD:
P1: Farmer's Carry: 100ft -
#90/#70
P2: AbMat Sit Up (Score)
P3: Burpee
AMRAP: 10 Minutes

LIFTING/SKILL DEV:
Rope Climb Skills

SKILL/DEV. WORK:
NOTE: GAMES TRACK DO THIS
Row: 5k (Recover and Stretch)
Ankles Up

190

WEEK 28 -
SAT FEB 11 2012

PHASE I:
Games Track Athletes - All

WARMUP:
4 Rounds of
:15 Jumping Jack
:15 Squat
:15 Mountain Climber
:15 Jump Squat
Then
30/20/30

EQUIPMENT:
BB #225/#155; Box 24/20

WOD:
Roy
DL: 15
Box Jump: 20
Pull Up: 25
5 Rounds for time

GAMES WOD:
Swing: 12-12-12-12-12
EMOTM (#124/#88)

ACCESSORY:
Olympic Weightlifting

Week 29

	SUNDAY 2/12	MONDAY 2/13	TUESDAY 2/14
WARM UP	**4 Rounds of** :15 Jumping Jack :15 Squat :15 MC :15 Jump Squat	Run/Lunge 3x Run/Bear Crawl 3x Run/Inchworm 3x Run: Broad Jump 3x	**4 Rounds of** :15 Jumping Jack :15 Squat :15 MC :15 Jump Squat
EQUIPMENT		BB: #315/205	BB #225/#155
WOD	Burpee: 12 Pull Up: 12 *5 Rounds for time*	DL: 2 *EMOTM for 10 Minutes*	FSQ: 2 *EMOTM for 10 Minutes*
LIFTING/SKILL	TGU: 1R/1L - *AMRAP: 12 Minutes*	*Partner KB Ladder w/(2 x 24/16kg) 1, 2, 3, 4, …?? For 15 Minutes*	Low Box Jump: Max Reps for :30 -*Rest :30 - 10 Minutes*
GAMES Phase I	Rest	All	All
SKILL/DEV WORK		MU Transition: 10 DHPU: 10 Dip: 10 Ring Dips: 10 MU (Strict): 10 HSPU: 10 L-Sit - :20/:10 x 8 Rope Climbs: 5	TGU: 1R/1L x 10 Run: 400 x 6 - *Rest 1:00* Hand Walk: 40ft *Note: Sub wall walk: if no hand walk (15)*
GAMES WOD		Run: 1 Mile - *Rest 5:00 - 4 Rounds*	Swing: 12-12-12-12-12 *EMOTM #124/#88*
ACCESSORY			

NOTES

192

WEDNESDAY 2/15	THURSDAY 2/16	FRIDAY 2/17	SATURDAY 2/18
Run/Lunge 3x Run/Bear Crawl 3x Run/Inchworm 3x Run: Broad Jump 3x	**4 Rounds of** :15 Jumping Jack :15 Squat :15 MC :15 Jump Squat	Run/Lunge 3x Run/Bear Crawl 3x Run/Inchworm 3x Run: Broad Jump 3x	**4 Rounds of** :15 Jumping Jack :15 Squat :15 MC :15 Jump Squat
BB: #315/205	BB #275/185		
SDL: 2 *EMOTM for 10 Minutes*	BSQ: 2 *EMOTM for 10 Minutes*	Pull Up: 10 Push Up: 20 Squat: 30 *AMRAP: 20 Minutes*	*Randy*
7 Rounds of Pull up: 7 Swing: 7 (24/16) Slam: 7 (30/20)	Box Jump: 7 (24/16) *EMOTM for 10 Minutes*	*Instructor Games*	
All	**All**	**Rest**	**All**
MU Transition: 10 DHPU: 10 Dip: 10 Ring Dips: 10 MU (Strict): 10 HSPU: 10 L-Sit - :20/:10 x 8 Rope Climbs: 5	TGU: 1R/1L x 10 Run: 400 x 6 - *Rest 1:00* Hand Walk: 40ft *Note: Sub wall walk: if no hand walk (15)*	Row: 5k (Recover & Stretch) Ankles up	
Row 2,000 - *Rest 5:00 -* *4 Rounds*	Swing: 12-12-12-12-12 *EMOTM #124/#88*		Swing: 12-12-12-12-12 *EMOTM #124/#88*
Olympic Lifting			*Olympic Lifting*

NOTES

_____

_____

_____

_____

WEEK 29 -
SUN FEB 12 2012

PHASE I:
Games Track Athletes - Rest

WARMUP:
:15 Jumping Jack
:15 Squat
:15 Mountain Climber
:15 Jump Squat

WOD:
Burpee: 12
Pull Up: 12
5 Rounds for time

LIFTING/SKILL DEV:
TGU 1/1 - AMRAP: 12 Minutes

WEEK 29 -
MON FEB 13 2012

PHASE I:
Games Track Athletes - All

WARMUP:
Run/Lunge 3x
Run/Bear Crawl 3x
Run/Inchworm 3x
Run: Broad Jump 3x

EQUIPMENT: BB: #315/205

WOD:
DL: 2 EMOTM for 10 Minutes
LIFTING/SKILL DEV:
Partner KB Ladder (2) 24/16kg
1, 2, 3, 4, …?? For 15 Minutes

SKILL/DEV. WORK:
MU Transitions: 10
DHPU: 10
Dip: 10
Ring Dips: 10
MU (Strict): 10
HSPU: 10
L-Sit - :20/:10 x 8
Rope Climbs: 5

GAMES WOD:
Run: 1 Mile - Rest 5:00 -
4 Rounds

194

WEEK 29 - TUE FEB 14 2012

PHASE I:
Games Track Athletes - All

WARMUP:
:15 Jumping Jack
:15 Squat
:15 Mountain Climber
:15 Jump Squat

EQUIPMENT: BB #225/#155

WOD:
FSQ: 2 EMOTM 10 Minutes

LIFTING/SKILL DEV:
Low Box Jump: Max Reps for
:30 - :30 Rest - 10 Minutes

SKILL/DEV. WORK:
TGU: 1/1 x 10
Run: 400 x 6 - 1:00 Rest
Hand Walk: 40ft
Note: Sub wall walk:
if no hand walk (15)

GAMES WOD:
Swing: 12-12-12-12-12
EMOTM (#124/#88)

WEEK 29 - WED FEB 15 2012

PHASE I:
Games Track Athletes - All

WARMUP:
Run/Lunge 3x
Run/Bear Crawl 3x
Run/Inchworm 3x
Run: Broad Jump 3x

EQUIPMENT: BB: #315/205

WOD:
SDL: 2 EMOTM for 10 Minutes

LIFTING/SKILL DEV:
7 Rounds of
Pull up: 7
Swing: 7 (24/16)
Slam: 7 (30/20)

SKILL/DEV. WORK:
MU Transitions: 10
DHPU: 10
Dip: 10
Ring Dips: 10
MU (Strict): 10
HSPU: 10
L-Sit - :20/:10 x 8
Rope Climbs: 5

GAMES WOD:
Row: 2,000 - Rest 5:00 -
4 Rounds

ACCESSORY:
Olympic Lifting

WEEK 29 -
THU FEB 16 2012

PHASE I:
Games Track Athletes - All

WARMUP:
:15 Jumping Jack
:15 Squat
:15 Mountain Climber
:15 Jump Squat

EQUIPMENT: BB #275/185

WOD:
BSQ: 2 EMOTM for 10 Minutes

LIFTING/SKILL DEV:
Box Jump: 7 (24/16) EMOTM
for 10 Minutes

SKILL/DEV. WORK:
TGU: 1/1 x 10
Run: 400 x 6 - 1:00 Rest
Hand Walk: 40ft
Note: Sub wall walk:
if no hand walk (15)

GAMES WOD:
Swing: 12-12-12-12-12
EMOTM (#124/#88)

WEEK 29 -
FRI FEB 17 2012

PHASE I:
Games Track Athletes - Rest

WARMUP:
Run/Lunge 3x
Run/Bear Crawl 3x
Run/Inchworm 3x
Run: Broad Jump 3x

WOD:
Pull Up: 10
Push Up: 20
Squat: 30
AMRAP: 20 Minutes

LIFTING/SKILL DEV:
Instructor Games

SKILL/DEV. WORK:
Row: 5k (Recover & Stretch)
Ankles up

WEEK 29 -
SAT FEB 18 2012

PHASE I:
Games Track Athletes - All

WARMUP:
:15 Jumping Jack
:15 Squat
:15 Mountain Climber
:15 Jump Squat

WOD:
Randy

GAMES WOD:
Swing: 12-12-12-12-12
EMOTM (#124/#88)

ACCESSORY:
Olympic Lifting

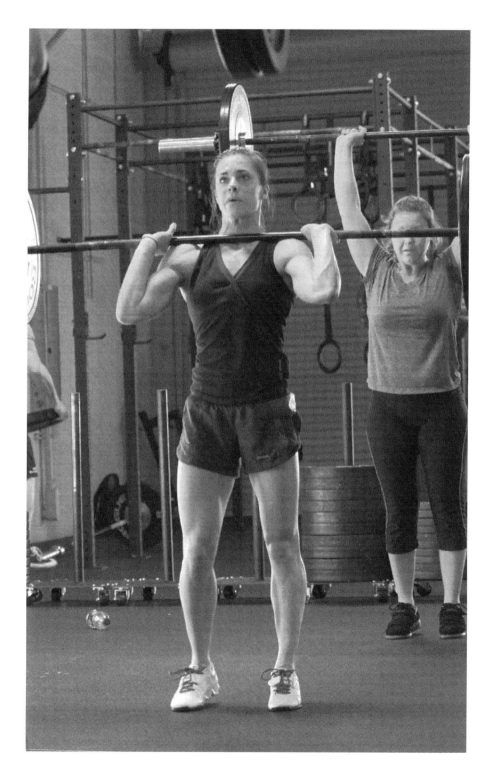

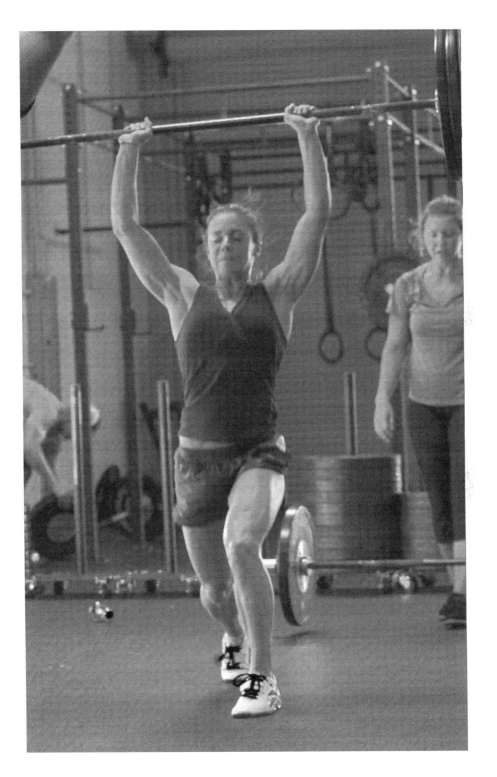

Week 30

	SUNDAY 2/19	MONDAY 2/20	TUESDAY 2/21
WARM UP	*Tabata* Style - : *20/:10 x 24 Intervals* Jumping Jack Squat MC Jump Squat	Run/Lunge 2x Run/Bear Crawl 2x Run/Inchworm 2x Run/Cartwheel 2x Run/Crabwalk 2x Low Box Jump :30/:30 x 5	*5 Rounds of* Jumping Jack 1:00 Squat Hold 1:00
EQUIPMENT	BB 155/105	Box 24/20	DB: (2) 35 BB: 225/155
WOD	DL: 1 CL: 1 FSQ: 1 J: 1 *AMRAP: 20 Minutes*	Box Jump: 12 Pull Up: 10 *5 Rounds for time*	Thruster: 7 Deadlift: 12 *3 Rounds for time*
LIFTING/SKILL	Roll and Recover	BSQ: 5-5-5-5-5 *EMOTM* @80% of 1RM	FSQ: 5-5-5-5-5 *EMOTM* @80% of 1RM
GAMES Phase I	Rest	All	All
SKILL/DEV WORK		MU Transition: 10 DHPU: 10 Dip: 10 Ring Dips: 10 Ring Row (Strict): 10 MU (Strict): 10 HSPU: 10 L-Sit - :20/:10 x 8 Rope Climbs: 5	TGU: 1R/1L x 5 Run: 800 x 4 - *Rest 1:00* Hand Walk: 40ft *Note: Sub wall walk: if no hand walk (15)* Weighted Pull Up: 5 x 5-*Kip or otherwise*
GAMES WOD		SN: 5 (135/95) Burpee: 12 *5 Rounds for time*	Row: 250M -*Rest 1:00* - 10 *Rounds*
ACCESSORY		Swing: 12-12-12-12-12 *EMOTM #124/#88*	Swing: 12-12-12-12-12 *EMOTM #124/#88*

NOTES

200

WEDNESDAY 2/22	THURSDAY 2/23	FRIDAY 2/24	SATURDAY 2/25
Run/Lunge 2x Run/Bear Crawl 2x Run/Inchworm 2x Run/Cartwheel 2x Run/Crabwalk 2x Low Box Jump :30/:30 x 5	*Tabata Style - :20/ :10 x 24 Intervals* Jumping Jack Squat MC Jump Squat	Run/Lunge 2x Run/Bear Crawl 2x Run/Inchworm 2x Run/Cartwheel 2x Run/Crabwalk 2x Low Box Jump :30/:30 x 5 **Then** *SPECIAL*	*TBA*
BB: 115/75	Ball: 30/20 BB 95/65	Dynamax: 20/14	*TBA*
PSN: 8 T2B: 8 Ring Push Up: 8 *AMRAP: 8 Minutes*	Row: 1,000 Double Unders: 90 AbMat SU: 80 Push Up (HR): 70 Ball Slam: 60 HPCL: 50 PP: 40 PJ: 30 Burpee: 20 Pull Up: 10 *For time*	**A1** : Row: 250 (Pace) **A2** : Wall Ball (score) **A3** : Push Up (score) *AMRAP: 12 Minutes*	*Games Open 12.1*
DL: 5-5-5-5-5 *EMOTM* @80% of 1RM	Roll and Recover	Roll and Recover	
All	**All**	**Active Rest**	**All**
MU Transition: 10 DHPU: 10 Dip: 10 Ring Dips: 10 Ring Row (Strict): 10 MU (Strict): 10 HSPU: 10 L-Sit - :20/:10 x 8 Rope Climbs: 5		Row: 3K Roll and Recover	
			Swing: 12-12-12-12-12 *EMOTM*
Olympic Lifting			*Olympic Lifting*

NOTES

WEEK 30 -
SUN FEB 19 2012

PHASE I:
Games Track Athletes - Rest

WARMUP:
Tabata Style -
:20/:10 x 24 Intervals
Jumping Jack
Squat
Mountain Climber
Jump Squat

EQUIPMENT: BB 155/105

WOD:
DL: 1
CL: 1
FSQ: 1
J: 1
AMRAP: 20 Minutes

LIFTING/SKILL DEV:
Roll and Recover

WEEK 30 -
MON FEB 20 2012

PHASE I:
Games Track Athletes - All

WARMUP:
Run/Lunge 2x
Run/Bear Crawl 2x
Run/Inchworm 2x
Run/Cartwheel 2x
Run/Crabwalk 2x
Then
Low Box Jump :30/:30 x 5

EQUIPMENT: Box 24/20

WOD:
Box Jump: 12
Pull Up: 10
5 Rounds for time

LIFTING/SKILL DEV:
BSQ: 5-5-5-5-5 EMOTM

SKILL/DEV. WORK:
MU Transitions: 10
DHPU: 10
Dip: 10
Ring Dips: 10
Ring Row: 10 (Strict)
MU (Strict): 10
HSPU: 10
L-Sit - :20/:10 x 8
Rope Climbs: 5

GAMES WOD:
SN: 5 (135/95)
Burpee: 12
5 Rounds for time

ACCESSORY:
Swing: 12-12-12-12-12
EMOTM (#124/#88)

WEEK 30 - TUE FEB 21 2012

PHASE I:
Games Track Athletes - All

WARMUP:
5 Rounds of
Jumping Jack: 1:00
Squat Hold: 1:00

EQUIPMENT:
DB: (2) 35; BB: 225/155

WOD:
Thruster: 7
Deadlift: 12
3 Rounds for time

LIFTING/SKILL DEV:
FSQ: 5-5-5-5-5 EMOTM

SKILL/DEV. WORK:
TGU: 1/1 x 5
Run: 800 x 4 - 1:00 Rest
Hand Walk: 40ft
Note: Sub wall walk:
if no hand walk (15)
Weighted Pull Up: 5 x 5 -
Kip or otherwise

GAMES WOD:
Row: 250M - Rest 1:00 -
10 Rounds

ACCESSORY:
Swing: 12-12-12-12-12
EMOTM (#124/#88)

WEEK 30 - WED FEB 22 2012

PHASE I:
Games Track Athletes - All

WARMUP:
Run/Lunge 2x
Run/Bear Crawl 2x
Run/Inchworm 2x
Run/Cartwheel 2x
Run/Crabwalk 2x
Then
Low Box Jump :30/:30 x 5

EQUIPMENT: BB: 115/75

WOD:
PSN: 8
T2B: 8
Ring Push Up: 8
AMRAP: 8 Minutes

LIFTING/SKILL DEV:
DL: 5-5-5-5-5 EMOTM

SKILL/DEV. WORK:
MU Transitions: 10
DHPU: 10
Dip: 10
Ring Dips: 10
Ring Row: 10 (Strict)
MU (Strict): 10
HSPU: 10
L-Sit - :20/:10 x 8
Rope Climbs: 5

ACCESSORY:
Olympic Lifting

WEEK 30 -
THU FEB 23 2012

PHASE I:
Games Track Athletes - All

WARMUP:
Tabata Style -
:20/:10 x 24 Intervals
Jumping Jack
Squat
Mountain Climber
Jump Squat

EQUIPMENT:
Ball: 30/20; BB 95/65

WOD:
Row: 1,000
Double Unders: 90
AbMat SU: 80
Push Up: 70 (HR)
Ball Slam: 60
HPCL: 50
PP: 40
PJ: 30
Burpee: 20
Pull Up: 10
For time

LIFTING/SKILL DEV:
Roll and recover

WEEK 30 -
FRI FEB 24 2012

PHASE I:
Games Track Athletes -
Active Rest

WARMUP:
Run/Lunge 2x
Run/Bear Crawl 2x
Run/Inchworm 2x
Run/Cartwheel 2x
Run/Crabwalk 2x
Low Box Jump :30/:30 x 5
Then
Special

EQUIPMENT:
Dynamax: 20/14

WOD:
P1: Row: 250 (Pace)
P2: Wall Ball (score)
P3: Push Up (score)
AMRAP: 12 Minutes

LIFTING/SKILL DEV:
Roll and recover

SKILL/DEV. WORK:
Row: 3K
Roll and recover

WEEK 30 -
SAT FEB 25 2012

PHASE I:
Games Track Athletes - All

WARMUP:
TBA

EQUIPMENT:
TBA

WOD:
Games Open 12.1

GAMES WOD:
Swing: 12-12-12-12-12
EMOTM (#124/#88)

ACCESSORY:
Olympic Lifting

Week 31

	SUNDAY 2/26	MONDAY 2/27	TUESDAY 2/28
WARM UP	*Tabata* Style - : *20/:10 x 24 Intervals* Jumping Jack Squat MC Jump Squat	Run/Lunge 2x Run/Bear Crawl 2x Run/Inchworm 2x Run/Cartwheel 2x Run/Crabwalk 2x Low Box Jump :30/:30 x 5	*5 Rounds of* Jumping Jack 1:00 Squat Hold 1:00
EQUIPMENT	BB: 135/95	BB: 155/105	KB: 24/16 Box: 24/20
WOD	*Partner Grace* - 1/1 until both reach 30 Reps - *Squat* *Clean*	Push Jerk: 9 FSQ: 9 Pull Up: 9 *AMRAP: 9 Minutes*	Row: 500 **Then** American Swing Box Jump 21, 15, 9 for time
LIFTING/SKILL	*Tabata* - :20/:10 x 8 - *Rest 1:00* Squat Push Up Burpee	DL: 3-3-3-3-3 *EMOTM* @90% of 1RM	BSQ: 3-3-3-3-3 *EMOTM* @90% of 1RM
GAMES Phase I	Rest	All	All
SKILL/DEV WORK		MU Transition: 10 DHPU: 10 Dip: 10 Ring Dips: 10 Ring Row (Strict): 10 MU (Strict): 10 HSPU: 10 L-Sit - :20/:10 x 8 Rope Climbs: 5	TGU: 1R/1 L x 5 Run: 800 x 4 - *Rest 1:00* Hand Walk: 40ft *Note: Sub wall walk: if no hand walk (15)* Weighted Pull Up: 5 x 5 - *Kip or otherwise*
GAMES WOD		*Cluster EMOTM 12 Minutes* (build to heavy)	Butcher HiPush: 40ft (#70/#50) HSPU: 5 *AMRAP: 10 Minutes*
ACCESSORY		Swing: 12-12-12-12-12 *EMOTM #124/#88*	Swing: 12-12-12-12-12 *EMOTM #124/#88*

NOTES

206

WEDNESDAY 2/29	THURSDAY 3/1	FRIDAY 3/2	SATURDAY 3/3
Run/Lunge 2x Run/Bear Crawl 2x Run/Inchworm 2x Run/Cartwheel 2x Run/Crabwalk 2x Low Box Jump :30/:30 x 5	*Tabata Style - :20/ :10 x 24 Intervals* Jumping Jack Squat MC Jump Squat	Run/Lunge 2x Run/Bear Crawl 2x Run/Inchworm 2x Run/Cartwheel 2x Run/Crabwalk 2x Low Box Jump :30/:30 x 5	*TBA*
KB (2) 24/16	BB *Loading Variable Get heavy*	DB: (2): 30/20	*TBA*
KB FSQ: 15 Burpee: 12 T2B: 9 *AMRAP: 12 Minutes*	CL&J *EMOTM for 20 Minutes*	Lunge (High Carry): 40ft Push Press: 12 Bent Over Row: 12 *AMRAP: 15 Minutes*	*Games Open 12.2*
FSQ: 3-3-3-3-3 *EMOTM* @90% of 1RM	Roll and Recover	TGU: 1R/1 L - *AMRAP: 10 Minutes*	
All	**All**	**Active Rest**	**All**
MU Transition: 10 DHPU: 10 Dip: 10 Ring Dips: 10 Ring Row: 10 (Strict) MU (Strict): 10 HSPU: 10 L-Sit - :20/:10 x 8 Rope Climbs: 5		Row: 5k (Recover & Stretch)	
			Swing: 12-12-12-12-12 *EMOTM #124/#88*
Olympic Lifting			*Olympic Lifting*

NOTES

_____

_____

_____

WEEK 31 -
SUN FEB 26 2012

PHASE I:
Games Track Athletes - All

WARMUP:
Tabata Style -
:20/:10 x 24 Intervals
Jumping Jack
Squat
Mountain Climber
Jump Squat

EQUIPMENT:
BB: 135/95

WOD:
Partner Grace -
1/1 until both reach 30 Reps -
Squat Clean

LIFTING/SKILL DEV:
Tabata - :20/:10 x 8 -
1:00 Rest
Squat
Push Up
Burpee

WEEK 31 -
MON FEB 27 2012

PHASE I:
Games Track Athletes - All

WARMUP:
Run/Lunge 2x
Run/Bear Crawl 2x
Run/Inchworm 2x
Run/Cartwheel 2x
Run/Crabwalk 2x
Run/Spidey 2x
Low Box Jump :30/:30 x 5

EQUIPMENT: BB: 155/105

WOD:
Push Jerk: 9
FSQ: 9
Pull Up: 9
AMRAP: 9 Minutes

LIFTING/SKILL DEV:
DL: 3-3-3-3-3 EMOTM

SKILL/DEV. WORK:
MU Transitions: 10
DHPU: 10
Dip: 10
Ring Dips: 10
Ring Row: 10 (Strict)
MU (Strict): 10
HSPU: 10
L-Sit - :20/:10 x 8
Rope Climbs: 5

GAMES WOD:
Cluster EMOTM - 12 Minutes
(build to heavy)

ACCESSORY:
Swing: 12-12-12-12-12
EMOTM (#124/#88)

208

WEEK 31 - TUE FEB 28 2012

PHASE I:
Games Track Athletes - All

WARMUP:
5 Rounds of
Jumping Jack: 1:00
Squat Hold: 1:00

EQUIPMENT:
KB: 24/16; Box: 24/20

WOD:
Row: 500
Then
American Swing
Box Jump
21, 15, 9 for time

LIFTING/SKILL DEV:
BSQ: 3-3-3-3-3 EMOTM

SKILL/DEV. WORK:
TGU: 1/1 x 5
Run: 800 x 4 - 1:00 Rest
Hand Walk: 40ft
Note: Sub wall walk:
if no hand walk (15)
Weighted Pull Up: 5 x 5 -
Kip or otherwise

GAMES WOD:
Butcher Push: 40ft
HSPU: 5
AMRAP: 10 Minutes

ACCESSORY:
Swing: 12-12-12-12-12
EMOTM (#124/#88)

WEEK 31 - WED FEB 29 2012

PHASE I:
Games Track Athletes - All

WARMUP:
Run/Lunge 2x
Run/Bear Crawl 2x
Run/Inchworm 2x
Run/Cartwheel 2x
Run/Crabwalk 2x
Run/Spidey 2x
Low Box Jump :30/:30 x 5

EQUIPMENT:
KB (2) 24/16

WOD:
KB FSQ: 15
Burpee: 12
T2B: 9
AMRAP: 12 Minutes

LIFTING/SKILL DEV:
FSQ: 3-3-3-3-3 EMOTM

SKILL/DEV. WORK:
MU Transitions: 10
DHPU: 10
Dip: 10
Ring Dips: 10
Ring Row: 10 (Strict)
MU (Strict): 10
HSPU: 10
L-Sit - :20/:10 x 8
Rope Climbs: 5

ACCESSORY:
Olympic Lifting

WEEK 31 -
THU MAR 01 2012

PHASE I:
Games Track Athletes - All

WARMUP:
Tabata Style -
:20/:10 x 24 Intervals
Jumping Jack
Squat
Mountain Climber
Jump Squat

EQUIPMENT:
BB (Loading Variable) -
Get heavy

WOD:
CL&J EMOTM for 20 Minutes

LIFTING/SKILL DEV:
Roll and recover

WEEK 31 -
FRI MAR 02 2012

PHASE I:
Games Track Athletes - Active Rest

WARMUP:
Run/Lunge 2x
Run/Bear Crawl 2x
Run/Inchworm 2x
Run/Cartwheel 2x
Run/Crabwalk 2x
Run/Spidey 2x
Low Box Jump :30/:30 x 5

EQUIPMENT:
DB: (2): 30/20

WOD:
Lunge: 40ft (High Carry)
Push Press: 12
Bent Over Row: 12
AMRAP: 15 Minutes

LIFTING/SKILL DEV:
TGU 1/1 - AMRAP: 10 Minutes

SKILL/DEV. WORK:
Row: 5k (Recover & Stretch)

WEEK 31 -
SAT MAR 03 2012

PHASE I:
Games Track Athletes - All

WARMUP:
TBA

EQUIPMENT: TBA

WOD:
Games Open 12.2

GAMES WOD:
Swing: 12-12-12-12-12
EMOTM (#124/#88)

ACCESSORY:
Olympic Lifting

Week 32

	SUNDAY 3/4	MONDAY 3/5	TUESDAY 3/6
WARM UP	Run/Lunge: 2x Run/Bear Crawl: 2x Run/Crab Walk 2x Run/Power Skip 2x Run/Heel Kicks 2x Run/Straight Leg March 2x Run/Cartwheel 2x 30/20/30	**4 Rounds of** :15 Jumping Jack :15 Squat :15 MC :15 Jump Squat **Then** Jump Rope 5:00 - *Work on Double Unders*	Run/Lunge: 2x Run/Bear Crawl: 2x Run/Crab Walk 2x Run/Power Skip 2x Run/Heel Kicks 2x Run/Straight Leg March 2x Run/Cartwheel 2x 30/20/30
EQUIPMENT		BB: 95/65 Ball: 30/20 Box: 24/16	Jump Rope
WOD	*Partner WOD* Burpee 1-10 x1 Ring Row: 1-10 x1 Ring Push Up 1-10 x1 Pull Up 1-10 x1 *For time*	Thruster: 12 Ball Slam: 12 Box Jump: 12 *AMRAP: 12 Minutes*	Burpee: 15 Double Under: 30 *AMRAP: 15 Minutes*
LIFTING/SKILL		DL: 1-1-1-1-1-1-1 *EMOTM* @90% of 1RM	BSQ: 1-1-1-1-1-1-1 *EMOTM* @90% of 1RM
GAMES Phase I	Rest	All	All
SKILL/DEV WORK		MU (1 Transition + 1 Dip): 10 DHPU: 10 Dip: 10 Ring Dips: 10 MU (Strict: 1 MU+ 2 Dips): 10 HSPU: 10 L-Sit - :20/:10 x 8 Rope Climbs: 5	TGU: 1R/1 L x 10 Run: 400 x 6 - *Rest 1:00* Hand Walk: 40ft *Note: Sub wall walk: if no* *hand walk (15)* Parallette HSPU: 3-3-3-3-3
GAMES WOD			Swing: 12-12-12-12-12 *EMOTM #124/#88*
ACCESSORY			

NOTES

WEDNESDAY 3/7	THURSDAY 3/8	FRIDAY 3/9	SATURDAY 3/10
4 Rounds of :15 Jumping Jack :15 Squat :15 MC :15 Jump Squat **Then** Jump Rope 5:00 - *Work on Double Unders*	Run/Lunge: 2x Run/Bear Crawl: 2x Run/Crab Walk 2x Run/Power Skip 2x Run/Heel Kicks 2x Run/Straight Leg March 2x Run/Cartwheel 2x 30/20/30	**4 Rounds of** :15 Jumping Jack :15 Squat :15 MC :15 Jump Squat **Then** Jump Rope 5:00 - *Work on* *Double Unders*	*TBA*
Dynamax: #20/#14 KB 24/16kg	BB: 135/95		
Wall Ball: 15 Swing: 15 Push Up (HR): 15 *AMRAP: 8 Minutes*	*The Chief* PCL: 3 Push Up: 6 Squat: 9 *AMRAP: 3 Minutes - Rest* *1:00*	*Cindy*	*Games Open 12.3*
FSQ: 1-1-1-1-1-1-1 *EMOTM* @90% of 1RM	Roll and Recover		
All	**All**	**Active Rest**	**All**
MU (1 Transition + 1 Dip):10 DHPU: 10 Dip: 10 Ring Dips: 10 MU (Strict: 1 MU+ 2 Dips):10 HSPU: 10 L-Sit - :20/:10 x 8 Rope Climbs: 5	TGU: 1R/1 L x 10 Run: 400 x 6 - *Rest 1:00* Hand Walk: 40ft *Note: Sub wall walk: if no* *hand walk (15)* Parallette HSPU: 3-3-3-3-3	Row: 5k (Recover & Stretch) Ankles up	
	Swing: 12-12-12-12-12 *EMOTM #124/#88*		Swing: 12-12-12-12-12 *EMOTM #124/#88*
Olympic Lifting			*Olympic Lifting*

NOTES

WEEK 32 -
SUN MAR 04 2012

PHASE I:
Games Track Athletes - Rest

WARMUP:
Run/Lunge 2x
Run/Bear Crawl: 2x
Run/Crab Walk 2x
Run/Power Skip 2x
Run/Heel Kicks 2x
Run/Straight Leg March 2x
Run/Cartwheel 2x
30/20/30

WOD:
Partner WOD
Burpee 1-10 x1
Ring Row: 1-10 x1
Ring Push Up 1-10 x1
Pull Up 1-10 x1
For time

WEEK 32 -
MON MAR 05 2012

PHASE I:
Games Track Athletes - All

WARMUP:
4 Rounds of
:15 Jumping Jack
:15 Squat
:15 Mountain Climber
:15 Jump Squat
Then
Jump Rope: 5:00 -
Work on Double Unders

EQUIPMENT:
BB: 95/65; Ball: 30/20;
Box: 24/16

WOD:
Thruster: 12
Ball Slam: 12
Box Jump: 12
AMRAP: 12 Minutes

LIFTING/SKILL DEV:
DL: 1-1-1-1-1-1-1 EMOTM

SKILL/DEV. WORK:
MU Transitions: 1 + 1 Dip x 10
DHPU: 10
Dip: 10
Ring Dips: 10
MU (Strict): 1 + 2 Dips x 10
HSPU: 10
L-Sit - :20/:10 x 8
Rope Climbs: 5

WEEK 32 - TUE MAR 06 2012

PHASE I:
Games Track Athletes - All

WARMUP:
Run/Lunge: 2x
Run/Bear Crawl: 2x
Run/Crab Walk 2x
Run/Power Skip 2x
Run/Heel Kicks 2x
Run/Straight Leg March 2x
Run/Cartwheel 2x
30/20/30

EQUIPMENT: Jump Rope

WOD:
Burpee: 15
Double Under: 30
AMRAP: 15 Minutes

LIFTING/SKILL DEV:
BSQ: 1-1-1-1-1-1-1 EMOTM

SKILL/DEV. WORK:
TGU: 1/1 x 10
Run: 400 x 6 - 1:00 Rest
Hand Walk: 40ft
Note: Sub wall walk:
if no hand walk (15)
Parallette HSPU: 3-3-3-3-3

GAMES WOD:
Swing: 12-12-12-12-12
EMOTM (#124/#88)

WEEK 32 - WED MAR 07 2012

PHASE I:
Games Track Athletes - All

WARMUP:
4 Rounds of
:15 Jumping Jack
:15 Squat
:15 Mountain Climber
:15 Jump Squat
Then
Jump Rope: 5:00 -
Work on Double Unders

EQUIPMENT:
Dynamax: #20/#14;
KB 24/16kg

WOD:
Wall Ball: 15
Swing: 15
Push Up (HR): 15
AMRAP: 8 Minutes

LIFTING/SKILL DEV:
FSQ: 1-1-1-1-1-1-1 EMOTM

SKILL/DEV. WORK:
MU Transitions: 1 + 1 Dip x 10
DHPU: 10
Dip: 10
Ring Dips: 10
MU (Strict): 1 + 2 Dips x 10
HSPU: 10
L-Sit - :20/:10 x 8
Rope Climbs: 5

ACCESSORY:
Olympic Lifting

WEEK 32 -
THU MAR 08 2012

PHASE I:
Games Track Athletes - All

WARMUP:
Run/Lunge: 2x
Run/Bear Crawl: 2x
Run/Crab Walk 2x
Run/Power Skip 2x
Run/Heel Kicks 2x
Run/Straight Leg March 2x
Run/Cartwheel 2x
30/20/30

EQUIPMENT: BB: 135/95

WOD:
The Chief
PCL: 3
Push Up: 6
Squat: 9
AMRAP: 3:00 - 1:00 Rest -
5 Rounds

LIFTING/SKILL DEV:
Roll and recovery

SKILL/DEV. WORK:
TGU: 1/1 x 10
Run: 400 x 6 - 1:00 Rest
Hand Walk: 40ft
Note: Sub wall walk:
if no hand walk (15)
Parallette HSPU: 3-3-3-3-3

GAMES WOD:
Swing: 12-12-12-12-12
EMOTM (#124/#88)

WEEK 32 -
FRI MAR 09 2012

PHASE I:
Games Track Athletes -
Active Rest

WARMUP:
4 Rounds of
:15 Jumping Jack
:15 Squat
:15 Mountain Climber
:15 Jump Squat
Then
Jump Rope: 5:00 -
Work on Double Unders

WOD:
Cindy

SKILL/DEV. WORK:
Row: 5k (Recover & Stretch)
Ankles up

WEEK 32 -
SAT MAR 10 2012

PHASE I:
Games Track Athletes - All

WARMUP:
TBA

WOD:
Games Open 12.3

GAMES WOD:
Swing: 12-12-12-12-12
EMOTM (#124/#88)

ACCESSORY:
Olympic Lifting

Week 33

	SUNDAY 3/11	MONDAY 3/12	TUESDAY 3/13
WARM UP	**4 Rounds of** :30 Jump Rope :30 Plank Hold :30 Squat Hold **Then** :15 Jumping Jack :15 Squat :15 MC :15 Jump Squat	Run/Lunge: 2x Run/Bear Crawl: 2x Run/Crab Walk 2x Run/Power Skip 2x Run/Heel Kicks 2x Run/Straight Leg March 2x Run/Cartwheel 2x 30/20/30	**5 Rounds of** Jump Rope: 1:00 Squat Hold: 1:00 **Then w/BB** **4 Rounds of** Dip/Catch: 3 Dip/Catch/Squat: 3 CL: 3 SJ: 3
EQUIPMENT	Dynamax #20/#14	BB #275/185	Dynamax #20/#14
W O D	**A1** : Row: 200M **A2** : MBCL **A3** : K2E *AMRAP: 12 Minutes*	DL: 5 DU: 30 *AMRAP: 5 Minutes*	**4 Rounds of** Burpee: 9 Wall Ball: 12 *AMRAP: 4 Minutes -* *Rest 1:00*
LIFTING/SKILL	Rest and roll	Row: 2k *for time*	**5 Rounds of** Dip: 5 (Strict) Pull Up: 5 (Strict/weighted)
GAMES Phase I	Rest	All	All
SKILL/DEV WORK		MU (1 Transition +1 Dip):10 DHPU: 10 Dip: 10 Ring Dips: 10 MU(Strict:1MU+ 2 Dips):10 HSPU: 10 L-Sit - :20/:10 x 8 Rope Climbs: 5	TGU: 1R/1L x 5 Run: 400 x 6 - *Rest 1:00* Hand Walk: 40ft *Note: Sub wall walk: if no* *hand walk (15)*
GAMES W O D		CL: 5 (185/120) BSQ: 7 (#225/135) *AMRAP: 7 Minutes*	Swing: 12-12-12-12-12 *EMOTM #124/#88*
ACCESSORY			Sled Drag: 800 - 135/90 *time*
POWER HOUR @ 90% of 1RM		BSQ 2 Reps x 10 Sets PJ 2 Reps x 10 Sets	FSQ: 2 Reps x 10 Sets SJ 2 Reps x 10 Sets
Basic Strength @ 80% of 1RM		BSQ: 5-5-5-5-5 P: 5-5-5-5-5	DL: 5-5-5-5-5 OHS: 5-5-5-5-5

WEDNESDAY 3/14	THURSDAY 3/15	FRIDAY 3/16	SATURDAY 3/17
Run/Lunge: 2x Run/Bear Crawl: 2x Run/Crab Walk 2x Run/Power Skip 2x Run/Heel Kicks 2x Run/Straight Leg March 2x Run/Cartwheel 2x 30/20/30	**5 Rounds of** Jump Rope 1:00 Squat Hold 1:00 **Then 3 Rounds of** MSCL: 3 MSCL-FSQ: 3 HCL: 3 **Then 3 Rounds of** Jerk Balance: 3 (Stagger) Jerk from Split: 3 Punch Under Drill: 3 SJ: 3	**4 Rounds of** :30 Jump Rope :30 Plank Hold :30 Squat Hold **Then** :15 Jumping Jack :15 Squat :15 MC :15 Jump Squat	Run: 400 30/20/30
BB: 155/100	BB *Load progressively*	DB: #30/#20	
DT DL: 12 HPCL: 9 PJ: 6 *5 Rounds for time*	CL+FSQ+SJ *EMOTM for 20 Minutes*	Thruster: 10 Walking Lunge (High Carry): 40ft Push Press: 10 *AMRAP: 12 Minutes*	*Games Open 12.4*
Rest and roll	Rest and Roll	Rest and Roll	
All	**All**	**Active Rest**	**All**
MU (1 Transition +1 Dip):10 DHPU: 10 Dip: 10 Ring Dips: 10 MU (Strict:1 MU+ 2 Dips):10 HSPU: 10 L-Sit - :20/:10 x 8 Rope Climbs: 5		Row: 5k (Recover & Stretch) Ankles up	
Butcher Push: 50yds #180/120 Handle Carry 50yds #90/#70 *AMRAP: 12 Minutes*	Swing: 12-12-12-12-12 *EMOTM #124/#88*		Swing: 12-12-12-12-12 *EMOTM #124/#88*
Olympic Lifting			*Olympic Lifting*
DL: 2 Reps x 10 Sets			
FSQ: 5-5-5-5-5 PP: 5-5-5-5-5	Pull Up: 5-5-5-5-5 PJ: 5-5-5-5-5		

WEEK 33 - SUN MAR 11 2012

PHASE I:
Games Track Athletes - Rest

WARMUP:
4 Rounds of
:30 Jump Rope
:30 Plank Hold
:30 Squat Hold
Then
:15 Jumping Jack
:15 Squat
:15 Mountain Climber
:15 Jump Squat

EQUIPMENT:
Dynamax #20/#14

WOD:
P1: Row: 200M
P2: MBCL
P3: K2E
AMRAP: 12 Minutes

LIFTING/SKILL DEV:
Rest and roll

WEEK 33 - MON MAR 12 2012

PHASE I:
Games Track Athletes - All

WARMUP:
Run/Lunge: 2x
Run/Bear Crawl: 2x
Run/Crab Walk 2x
Run/Power Skip 2x
Run/Heel Kicks 2x
Run/Straight Leg March 2x
Run/Cartwheel 2x
30/20/30

EQUIPMENT: BB #275/185

WOD:
DL: 5
DU: 30
AMRAP: 5 Minutes

LIFTING/SKILL DEV:
Row: 2k for time

SKILL/DEV. WORK:
MU Transitions: 1 + 1 Dip x 10
DHPU: 10
Dip: 10
Ring Dips: 10
MU (Strict): 1 + 2 Dips x 10
HSPU: 10
L-Sit - :20/:10 x 8
Rope Climbs: 5

GAMES WOD:
CL: 5 (185/120)
BSQ: 7 (#225/135)
AMRAP: 7 Minutes

POWER HOUR:
BSQ: 2 reps x 10 Sets
PJ: 2 reps x 10 Sets

BASIC STRENGTH:
BSQ: 5-5-5-5-5
P: 5-5-5-5-5

220

WEEK 33 -
TUE MAR 13 2012

PHASE I:
Games Track Athletes - All

WARMUP:
5 Rounds of
Jump Rope: 1:00
Squat Hold: 1:00
Then w/BB: Barbell Complex
4 Rounds of
Dip/Catch: 3
Dip/Catch/Squat: 3
CL: 3
SJ: 3

EQUIPMENT: Dynamax #20/#14

WOD:
Burpee: 9
Wall Ball: 12
AMRAP 4:00 - 1:00 Rest -
4 Rounds

LIFTING/SKILL DEV:
5 Rounds of
Dip: 5 (Strict)
Pull Up: 5 (Strict/weighted)

SKILL/DEV. WORK:
TGU: 1/1 x 5
Run: 400 x 6 - 1:00 Rest
Hand Walk: 40ft
Note: Sub wall walk:
if no hand walk (15)

GAMES WOD:
Swing: 12-12-12-12-12
EMOTM (#124/#88)

ACCESSORY:
Sled Drag: 800 (135/90) - for time

POWER HOUR:
FSQ: 2 reps x 10 Sets
SJ: 2 reps x 10 Sets

BASIC STRENGTH:
DL: 5-5-5-5-5
OHS: 5-5-5-5-5

WEEK 33 -
WED MAR 14 2012

PHASE I:
Games Track Athletes - All

WARMUP:
Run/Lunge: 2x
Run/Bear Crawl: 2x
Run/Crab Walk 2x
Run/Power Skip 2x
Run/Heel Kicks 2x
Run/Straight Leg March 2x
Run/Cartwheel 2x
30/20/30

EQUIPMENT: BB: 155/100

WOD:
DT
DL: 12
HPCL: 9
PJ: 6
5 Rounds for time

SKILL/DEV. WORK:
MU Transitions: 1 + 1 Dip x 10
DHPU: 10
Dip: 10
Ring Dips: 10
MU (Strict): 1 + 2 Dips x 10
HSPU: 10
L-Sit - :20/:10 x 8
Rope Climbs: 5

GAMES WOD:
Butcher Push: 50yds - #180/120
Handle Carry: 50yds - #90/#70
AMRAP: 12 Minutes

ACCESSORY:
Olympic Lifting

POWER HOUR:
DL: 2 reps x 10 Sets

BASIC STRENGTH:
FSQ: 5-5-5-5-5
PP: 5-5-5-5-5

221

WEEK 33 - THU MAR 15 2012

PHASE I:
Games Track Athletes - All

WARMUP:
5 Rounds of
Jump Rope: 1:00
Squat Hold: 1:00
Then 3 Rounds of
MSCL: 3
MSCL-FSQ: 3
HCL: 3
Then 3 Rounds of
Jerk Balance: 3 (Stagger)
Jerk from Split: 3
Punch Under Drill: 3
SJ: 3

EQUIPMENT:
BB - Load progressively

WOD:
CL+FSQ+SJ EMOTM for
20 Minutes

LIFTING/SKILL DEV:
Rest and roll

GAMES WOD:
Swing: 12-12-12-12-12
EMOTM (#124/#88)

BASIC STRENGTH:
Pull Up: 5-5-5-5-5
PJ: 5-5-5-5-5

WEEK 33 - FRI MAR 16 2012

PHASE I:
Games Track Athletes -
Active Rest

WARMUP:
4 Rounds of
:30 Jump Rope
:30 Plank Hold
:30 Squat Hold
Then
:15 Jumping Jack
:15 Squat
:15 Mountain Climber
:15 Jump Squat

EQUIPMENT: DB: #30/#20

WOD:
Thruster: 10
Walking Lunge (High Carry):
40ft
Push Press: 10
AMRAP: 12 Minutes

LIFTING/SKILL DEV:
Rest and roll

SKILL/DEV. WORK:
Row: 5k (Recover & Stretch)
Ankles up

WEEK 33 -
SAT MAR 17 2012

PHASE I:
Games Track Athletes - All

WARMUP:
Run: 400
30/20/30

WOD:
Games Open 12.4

GAMES WOD:
Swing: 12-12-12-12-12
EMOTM (#124/#88)

ACCESSORY:
Olympic Lifting

Week 34

	SUNDAY 3/18	MONDAY 3/19	TUESDAY 3/20
WARM UP	**4 Rounds of** :15 Jumping Jack :15 Squat :15 MC :15 Jump Squat **Then** 30/20/30	**4 Rounds of** :15 Jumping Jack :15 Squat :15 MC :15 Jump Squat **Then** 30/20/30	Run: 400 30/20/30
EQUIPMENT		KB 28kg/20kg	BB #135/95
WOD	**A1** : Run: 100 **A2** : Push Up (HR) (Score) **A3** : Squat (Score) **AMRAP: 12 Minutes**	American Swing: 30 Pull Up: 15 **3 Rounds for time**	Row: 1000 **Then** Push Jerk Power Clean BSQ **21, 15, 9 for time**
LIFTING/SKILL	*Dodgeball*	BSQ: 5 Reps x 5 Sets **EMOTM** @80% of 1RM	FSQ: 5 Reps x 5 Sets **EMOTM** @80% of 1RM
GAMES Phase I	Rest	All	All
SKILL/DEV WORK		MU Transition: 10 DHPU: 5-5-5-5-5 Dip: 5-5-5-5-5 Ring Dips: 5-5-5-5-5 MU (Kip): 3-3-3-3-3 HSPU: 3-3-3-3-3 L-Sit - :20/:10 x 8 Rope Climbs: 5	TGU: 1R/1L x 5 Run: 400 x 6 - **Rest 1:00** Hand Walk: 40ft **Note: Sub wall walk:** **if no hand walk (15)** KB FSQ 12-12-12-12-12 **EMOTM** (24kg/16kg)
GAMES WOD		CL&J - **Prison Rules** - 2 Reps every :15 x 16 (135/95)	Swing: 15-15-15-15-15 **EMOTM** #124/#88
ACCESSORY			

NOTES

WEDNESDAY 3/21	THURSDAY 3/22	FRIDAY 3/23	SATURDAY 3/24
Run: 400 30/20/30	**4 Rounds of** :15 Jumping Jack :15 Squat :15 MC :15 Jump Squat **Then** 30/20/30	Run: 400 30/20/30 **Then 4 Rounds of** :15 Jumping Jack :15 Squat :15 MC :15 Jump Squat	*TBA*
BB 120/75		DB (2): #35/#25 Slammer: #30/#20 Dynamax #20/#14	
Thruster: 7 Burpee: 7 **AMRAP: 7 Minutes**	*Tabata:*- :20/:10 x 8 - **Rest** **1:00** Squats Push Up (HR) AbMat Ball Slam	Weighted Step Ups R/L Ball Slam Wall Ball **21, 15, 9 for time**	*Gam*
All	**All**	**Rest**	**All**
CL&J - **Prison Rules** - 2 Reps every :15 x 16 (135/95)	Swing: 15-15-15-15-15 **EMOTM** #124/#88		Swing: 15-15-15-15-15 **EMOTM** #124/#88
Olympic Lifting			*Olympic Lifting*

NOTES

WEEK 34 -
SUN MAR 18 2012

PHASE I:
Games Track Athletes - Rest

WARMUP:
:15 Jumping Jack
:15 Squat
:15 Mountain Climber
:15 Jump Squat
30/20/30

WOD:
P1: Run: 100
P2: Push Up (HR) (Score)
P3: Squat (Score)

LIFTING/SKILL DEV:
Dodgeball

WEEK 34 -
MON MAR 19 2012

PHASE I:
Games Track Athletes - All

WARMUP:
:15 Jumping Jack
:15 Squat
:15 Mountain Climber
:15 Jump Squat
30/20/30

EQUIPMENT: KB 28kg/20kg

WOD:
American Swing: 30
Pull Up: 15
3 Rounds for time

LIFTING/SKILL DEV:
BSQ: 5 Reps EMOTM for
5 Sets

SKILL/DEV. WORK:
MU Transitions: 10
DHPU: 5-5-5-5-5
Dip: 5-5-5-5-5
Ring Dips: 5-5-5-5-5
MU (Kip): 3-3-3-3-3
HSPU: 3-3-3-3-3
L-Sit - :20/:10 x 8
Rope Climbs: 5

GAMES WOD:
CL&J - Prison Rules -
2 Reps every :15 x 16
(135/95)

WEEK 34 - TUE MAR 20 2012

PHASE I:
Games Track Athletes - All

WARMUP:
Run: 400
30/20/30

EQUIPMENT: BB #135/95

WOD:
Row: 1000
Then
Push Jerk
Power Clean
BSQ
21-15-9 for time

LIFTING/SKILL DEV:
FSQ: 5 Reps EMOTM for
5 sets

SKILL/DEV. WORK:
TGU: 1/1 x 5
Run: 400 x 6 - 1:00 Rest
Hand Walk: 40ft
Note: Sub wall walk:
if no hand walk (15)
KB FSQ 12-12-12-12-12
EMOTM (24kg/16kg)

GAMES WOD:
Swing: 15-15-15-15-15
EMOTM (#124/#88)

WEEK 34 - WED MAR 21 2012

PHASE I:
Games Track Athletes - All

WARMUP:
Run: 400
30/20/30

EQUIPMENT: BB 120/75

WOD:
Thruster: 7
Burpee: 7
AMRAP: 7 Minutes

LIFTING/SKILL DEV:
DL: 5 Reps EMOTM for
5 sets

SKILL/DEV. WORK:
MU Transitions: 10
DHPU: 10
Dip: 10
Ring Dips: 10
Ring Row: 10 (Strict)
MU: 10 (Strict)
HSPU: 10
L-Sit - :20/:10 x 8
Rope Climbs: 5

GAMES WOD:
CL&J - Prison Rules -
2 Reps every :15 x 16
(135/95)

ACCESSORY:
Olympic Lifting

WEEK 34 - THU MAR 22 2012

PHASE I:
Games Track Athletes - All

WARMUP:
:15 Jumping Jack
:15 Squat
:15 Mountain Climber
:15 Jump Squat
30/20/30

WOD:
Tabata - :20/:10 x 8 -
1:00 Rest
Squats
Push Up (HR)
AbMat
Ball Slam

LIFTING/SKILL DEV:
Roll and Rest

SKILL/DEV. WORK:
TGU: 1/1 x 5
Run: 400 x 6 - 1:00 Rest
Hand Walk: 40ft
Note: Sub wall walk:
if no hand walk (15)

GAMES WOD:
Swing: 15-15-15-15-15
EMOTM (#124/#88)

WEEK 34 - FRI MAR 23 2012

PHASE I:
Games Track Athletes - Rest

WARMUP:
Run: 400
30/20/30
:15 Jumping Jack
:15 Squat
:15 Mountain Climber
:15 Jump Squat

EQUIPMENT:
DB (2): #35/#25;
Slammer: #30/#20;
Dynamax #20/#14

WOD:
Weighted Step Ups R/L
Ball Slam
Wall Ball
21-15-9 for time

SKILL/DEV. WORK:
Row: 5k (Recover & Stretch)
Ankles up

WEEK 34 -
SAT MAR 24 2012

PHASE I:
Games Track Athletes - All

WARMUP:
TBA

WOD:
Games Open 12.5

GAMES WOD:
Swing: 15-15-15-15-15
EMOTM (#124/#88)

ACCESSORY:
Olympic Lifting

NOTES

Week 35

	SUNDAY 3/25	MONDAY 3/26	TUESDAY 3/27
WARM UP	**4 Rounds of** :15 Jumping Jack :15 Squat :15 MC :15 Jump Squat **Then** 30/20/30	**4 Rounds of** :15 Jumping Jack :15 Squat :15 MC :15 Jump Squat **Then** 30/20/30	Run: 400 30/20/30
EQUIPMENT	Box 24/20 Dynamax 20/14		BB 95/65
W O D	*Kelly*	*Cindy*	*Nancy*
LIFTING/SKILL		DL: 3 Reps x 5 Sets **EMOTM** @90% of 1RM	FSQ: 3 Reps x 5 Sets **EMOTM** @90% of 1RM
GAMES Phase I	Rest	All	All
SKILL/DEV WORK		MU Transition: 10 DHPU: 5-5-5-5-5 Dip: 5-5-5-5-5 Ring Dips: 5-5-5-5-5 MU (Kip): 3-3-3-3-3 HSPU: 3-3-3-3-3 L-Sit - :20/:10 x 8 Rope Climbs: 5	TGU: 1R/1L x 5 Run: 400 x 6 - **Rest 1:00** Hand Walk: 40ft **Note: Sub wall walk: if no hand walk (15)** KB FSQ 12-12-12-12-12 **EMOTM** (24kg/16kg)
GAMES W O D		CL&J -**Prison Rules** - 2 Reps every :15 x 16 (135/95)	Swing: 15-15-15-15-15 **EMOTM** #124/#88
ACCESSORY		GHD H&B Ext: 15 GHD Sit Up: 15 **3 Rounds (Completion)**	Thruster: 5 (BB 135/95) Muscle Up: 2 **AMRAP: 8 Minutes**

NOTES

_____

_____

_____

WEDNESDAY 3/28	THURSDAY 3/29	FRIDAY 3/30	SATURDAY 3/31
Run: 400 30/20/30	**4 Rounds of** :15 Jumping Jack :15 Squat :15 MC :15 Jump Squat **Then** 30/20/30	Run: 400 30/20/30 **Then 4 Rounds of** :15 Jumping Jack :15 Squat :15 MC :15 Jump Squat	*TBA*
BB 45/35			
Jackie	*McGhee*		
BSQ: 3 Reps x 5 Sets **EMOTM** @90% of 1RM			
All	**Rest**	**Active Rest**	**All**
MU Transition: 10 DHPU: 10 Dip: 10 Ring Dips: 10 Ring Row (Strict): 10 MU (Strict): 10 HSPU: 10 L-Sit - :20/:10 x 8 Rope Climbs: 5		Row: 5k (Recover & Stretch) Ankles up	*Murph*
CL&J - **Prison Rules** - 2 Reps every :15 x 16 (135/95)			
Olympic Lifting			*Olympic Lifting*

NOTES

_____

_____

_____

WEEK 35 -
SUN MAR 25 2012

PHASE I:
Games Track Athletes - Rest

WARMUP:
:15 Jumping Jack
:15 Squat
:15 Mountain Climber
:15 Jump Squat
30/20/30

EQUIPMENT:
Box 24/20; Dynamax 20/14

WOD:
Kelly

WEEK 35 -
MON MAR 26 2012

PHASE I:
Games Track Athletes - All

WARMUP:
:15 Jumping Jack
:15 Squat
:15 Mountain Climber
:15 Jump Squat
30/20/30

WOD:
Cindy

LIFTING/SKILL DEV:
DL: 3 Reps - 5 Sets
SKILL/DEV. WORK:
MU Transitions: 10
DHPU: 5-5-5-5-5
Dip: 5-5-5-5-5
Ring Dips: 5-5-5-5-5
MU (Kip): 3-3-3-3-3
HSPU: 3-3-3-3-3
L-Sit - :20/:10 x 8
Rope Climbs: 5

GAMES WOD:
CL&J - Prison Rules - 2 Reps
every :15 x 16 (135/95)

ACCESSORY:
GHD H&B Ext: 15
GHD Sit Up: 15
3 Rounds (Completion)

WEEK 35 - TUE MAR 27 2012

PHASE I:
Games Track Athletes - All

WARMUP:
Run: 400
30/20/30

EQUIPMENT: BB 95/65

WOD:
Nancy

LIFTING/SKILL DEV:
FSQ: 3 Reps - 5 Sets

SKILL/DEV. WORK:
TGU: 1/1 x 5
Run: 400 x 6 - 1:00 Rest
Hand Walk: 40ft
Note: Sub wall walk:
if no hand walk (15)
KB FSQ: 12-12-12-12-12
EMOTM (24kg/16kg)

GAMES WOD:
Swing: 15-15-15-15-15
EMOTM (#124/#88)

ACCESSORY:
Thruster: 5 (BB 135/95)
Muscle Up: 2
AMRAP: 8 Minutes

WEEK 35 - WED MAR 28 2012

PHASE I:
Games Track Athletes - All

WARMUP:
Run: 400
30/20/30

EQUIPMENT: BB 45/35

WOD:
Jackie

LIFTING/SKILL DEV:
BSQ: 3 Reps - 5 Sets

SKILL/DEV. WORK:
MU Transitions: 10
DHPU: 10
Dip: 10
Ring Dips: 10
Ring Row: 10 (Strict)
MU (Strict): 10
HSPU: 10
L-Sit - :20/:10 x 8
Rope Climbs: 5

GAMES WOD:
CL&J - Prison Rules - 2 Reps
every :15 x 16 (135/95)

ACCESSORY:
Olympic Lifting

233

**WEEK 35 -
THU MAR 29 2012**

PHASE I:
Games Track Athletes - Rest

WARMUP:
:15 Jumping Jack
:15 Squat
:15 Mountain Climber
:15 Jump Squat
30/20/30

WOD:
McGhee

**WEEK 35 -
FRI MAR 30 2012**

PHASE I:
Games Track Athletes -
Active Rest

WARMUP:
Run: 400
30/20/30
:15 Jumping Jack
:15 Squat
:15 Mountain Climber
:15 Jump Squat

SKILL/DEV. WORK:
Row: 5k (Recover & Stretch)
Ankles up

234

WEEK 35 -
SAT MAR 31 2012

PHASE I:
Games Track Athletes - All

WARMUP:
TBA

WOD:
Murph

ACCESSORY:
Olympic Lifting

Week 36

	SUNDAY 4/1	MONDAY 4/2	TUESDAY 4/3
WARM UP	Run: 400 30/20/30 **Then 4 Rounds of** :15 Jumping Jack :15 Squat :15 MC :15 Jump Squat **Then 4 Rounds of** :15 Plank :15 Superman :15 Side Plank /L :15 Side Plank /R	Run: 400 30/20/30 **Then 4 Rounds of** :15 Jumping Jack :15 Squat :15 MC :15 Jump Squat **Then 4 Rounds of** :15 Plank :15 Superman :15 Side Plank /L :15 Side Plank /R	Run: 400 30/20/30 **Then 4 Rounds of** :15 Jumping Jack :15 Squat :15 MC :15 Jump Squat **Then 4 Rounds of** :15 Plank :15 Superman :15 Side Plank /L :15 Side Plank /R
EQUIPMENT	KB: 24/16	Dynamax: 20/14 KB 28/20	Slammer: 30/20
WOD	**A1** : Run: 100 **A2** : Swing (Score) **A3** : Push Up (Score) **AMRAP: 12 Minutes**	Run: 200 Wall Ball: 20 Swing: 20 **AMRAP: 12 Minutes**	Ball Slam: 12 Burpee: 12 Toes to Bar: 12 **3 Rounds for time**
LIFTING/SKILL		FSQ: 2-2-2-2-2-2-2 **EMOTM** @90% of 1RM	BSQ: 2-2-2-2-2-2-2 **EMOTM** @90% of 1RM
GAMES Phase II	CAMP/All	**Active Rest**	**All**
SKILL/DEV WORK		Run: 5k (Recover & Stretch) Ankles up	TGU: 1R/1L x 5 Run: 400 x 6 - **Rest** **1:00** Hand Walk: 40ft **Note: Sub wall walk: if** **no hand walk (15)** KB FSQ 12-12-12-12-12 **EMOTM** (24kg/16kg)
GAMES WOD			Sprint: 100 Jog: 100 **AMRAP: 10 Minutes**
ACCESSORY			Swing: 15-15-15-15-15 **EMOTM** #124/#88
POWER HOUR **All lifts EMOTM** **@ 90% of 1RM**		Clean 2-2-2-2-2-2-2 Jerk/Blocks 2-2-2-2-2-2-2	SN: 2-2-2-2-2-2-2 PP: 2-2-2-2-2-2-2

WEDNESDAY 4/4	THURSDAY 4/5	FRIDAY 4/6	SATURDAY 4/7
Run: 400 30/20/30 **Then 4 Rounds of** :15 Jumping Jack :15 Squat :15 MC :15 Jump Squat **Then 4 Rounds of** :15 Plank :15 Superman :15 Side Plank /L :15 Side Plank /R	Run: 400 30/20/30 **Then 4 Rounds of** :15 Jumping Jack :15 Squat :15 MC :15 Jump Squat **Then 4 Rounds of** :15 Plank :15 Superman :15 Side Plank /L :15 Side Plank /R	Run: 400 30/20/30 **Then 4 Rounds of** :15 Jumping Jack :15 Squat :15 MC :15 Jump Squat **Then 4 Rounds of** :15 Plank :15 Superman :15 Side Plank /L :15 Side Plank /R	Run: 400 30/20/30 **Then 4 Rounds of** :15 Jumping Jack :15 Squat :15 MC :15 Jump Squat **Then 4 Rounds of** :15 Plank :15 Superman :15 Side Plank /L :15 Side Plank /R
BB: 95/65	BB: 135/95	BB 135/95	BB: 275/185 KB: 32/24 BB: 115/75 Box 24/20 DB 35/25
Run: 400 Thruster: 21 Ring Dip: 12 **3 Rounds for time**	BSQ: 12 Pull Up: 10 **4 Rounds for time**	*Grace* *(PCL)*	*Lumberjack: 20*
DL: 2-2-2-2-2-2-2 **EMOTM** @90% of 1RM	Row: 1k *for time*	*Dodgeball*	
All	**All**	**Active Rest**	**All**
MU Transition: 10 DHPU: 10 Dip: 10 Ring Dips: 10 Ring Row (Strict): 10 MU (Strict): 10 HSPU: 10 L-Sit - :20/:10 x 8 Rope Climbs: 5		Row: 5k (Recover & Stretch) Ankles up	Row: 500 - **Rest** **1:00 - 5 Rounds**
	Butcher HiPush: 25yds (90/70) Pistol 3R/3L **AMRAP: 12 Minutes**		Thruster 3-3-3-3-3-3-3
Olympic Lifting	CL&J - **Prison Rules** -2 Reps every :15 x16 (135/95)		*Olympic Lifting*
Sled Drag: 800 (135/90) **for time**	Sand Bag Carry: 25yds (#90/#70) Run: 50 **AMRAP: 10 Minutes**		

WEEK 36 - SUN APR 01 2012

PHASE I:
Games Track Athletes - All

WARMUP:
Run: 400
30/20/30
Then 4 Rounds of
:15 Jumping Jack
:15 Squat
:15 Mountain Climber
:15 Jump Squat
Then 4 Rounds of
:15 Plank
:15 Superman
:15 Side Plank - L
:15 Side Plank - R

EQUIPMENT: KB: 24/16

WOD:
P1: Run: 100
P2: Swing: (Score)
P3: Push Up (Score)
AMRAP: 12 minutes

GAMES: CAMP

WEEK 36 - MON APR 02 2012

PHASE II:
Games Track Athletes
- Active Rest

WARMUP:
Run: 400
30/20/30
Then 4 Rounds of
:15 Jumping Jack
:15 Squat
:15 Mountain Climber
:15 Jump Squat
Then 4 Rounds of
:15 Plank
:15 Superman
:15 Side Plank - L
:15 Side Plank - R

EQUIPMENT:
Dynamax: 20/14; KB 28/20

WOD:
Run: 200
Wall Ball: 20
Swing: 20
AMRAP: 12 Minutes

LIFTING/SKILL DEV:
FSQ: 2-2-2-2-2-2-2 EMOTM

SKILL/DEV. WORK:
Run: 5k (Recover & Stretch)
Ankles up

POWER HOUR:
Clean 2-2-2-2-2-2-2
Jerk from Blocks 2-2-2-2-2-2-2

238

WEEK 36 -
TUE APR 03 2012

PHASE II:
Games Track Athletes - All

WARMUP:
Run: 400
30/20/30
Then 4 Rounds of
:15 Jumping Jack
:15 Squat
:15 Mountain Climber
:15 Jump Squat
Then 4 Rounds of
:15 Plank
:15 Superman
:15 Side Plank - L
:15 Side Plank - R

EQUIPMENT: Slammer: 30/20

WOD:
Ball Slam: 12
Burpee: 12
Toes to Bar: 12
3 Rounds for time

LIFTING/SKILL DEV:
BSQ: 2-2-2-2-2-2-2 EMOTM

SKILL/DEV. WORK:
TGU: 1/1 x 5
Run: 400 x 6 - 1:00 Rest
Hand Walk: 40ft
Note: Sub wall walk:
if no hand walk (15)
KB FSQ: 12-12-12-12-12
EMOTM (24kg/16kg)

GAMES WOD:
Sprint: 100
Jog: 100
AMRAP: 10 Minutes

ACCESSORY:
Swing: 15-15-15-15-15 EMOTM
(#124/#88)

POWER HOUR:
SN: 2-2-2-2-2-2-2
PP: 2-2-2-2-2-2-2

WEEK 36 -
WED APR 04 2012

PHASE II:
Games Track Athletes - All

WARMUP:
Run: 400
30/20/30
Then 4 Rounds of
:15 Jumping Jack
:15 Squat
:15 Mountain Climber
:15 Jump Squat
Then 4 Rounds of
:15 Plank
:15 Superman
:15 Side Plank - L
:15 Side Plank - R

EQUIPMENT: BB: 95/65

WOD:
Run: 400
Thruster: 21
Ring Dip: 12
3 Rounds for time

LIFTING/SKILL DEV:
DL: 2-2-2-2-2-2-2 EMOTM

SKILL/DEV. WORK:
MU Transitions: 10
DHPU: 10
Dip: 10
Ring Dips: 10
Ring Row: 10 (Strict)
MU (Strict): 10
HSPU: 10
L-Sit - :20/:10 x 8
Rope Climbs: 5

ACCESSORY:
Olympic Lifting

POWER HOUR:
Sled Drag: 800 (135/90)
- for time

WEEK 36 - THU APR 05 2012

PHASE II:
Games Track Athletes - All

WARMUP:
Run: 400
30/20/30
Then 4 Rounds of
:15 Jumping Jack
:15 Squat
:15 Mountain Climber
:15 Jump Squat
Then 4 Rounds of
:15 Plank
:15 Superman
:15 Side Plank - L
:15 Side Plank - R

EQUIPMENT: BB: 135/95

WOD:
BSQ: 12
Pull Up: 10
4 Rounds for time

LIFTING/SKILL DEV:
Row: 1k for time

GAMES WOD:
Butcher Hi Push: 25yds
(90/70)
Pistol: 3R/3L
AMRAP: 12 Minutes

ACCESSORY:
CL&J - Prison Rules -
2 Reps every :15 x 16
(135/95)

POWER HOUR:
Sand Bag Carry: 25yds
(#90/#70)
Run: 50
AMRAP: 10 Minutes

WEEK 36 - FRI APR 06 2012

PHASE II:
Games Track Athletes -
Active Rest

WARMUP:
Run: 400
30/20/30
Then 4 Rounds of
:15 Jumping Jack
:15 Squat
:15 Mountain Climber
:15 Jump Squat
Then 4 Rounds of
:15 Plank
:15 Superman
:15 Side Plank - L
:15 Side Plank - R

EQUIPMENT: BB: 135/95

WOD:
Grace - PCL

LIFTING/SKILL DEV:
Dodgeball

SKILL/DEV. WORK:
Run: 5k
(Recover & Stretch)
Ankles up

WEEK 36 -
SAT APR 07 2012

PHASE II:
Games Track Athletes - All

WARMUP:
Run: 400
30/20/30
Then 4 Rounds of
:15 Jumping Jack
:15 Squat
:15 Mountain Climber
:15 Jump Squat
Then 4 Rounds of
:15 Plank
:15 Superman
:15 Side Plank - L
:15 Side Plank - R

EQUIPMENT:
BB: 275/185;
KG: 32/24;
BB: 115/75;
Box 24/20;
DB 35/25

WOD:
Lumberjack: 20

SKILL/DEV. WORK:
Row: 500 - Rest 1:00 - 5 Rounds

GAMES WOD:
Thruster 3-3-3-3-3-3-3

ACCESSORY:
Olympic Weightlifting

Week 37

	SUNDAY 4/8	MONDAY 4/9	TUESDAY 4/10
WARM UP	With empty bar 3 Rounds of DL: 3 PCL: 3 FSQ: 3 PJ: 3 OHS: 3	Run: 400 30/20/30 **Mobility: 10 Minutes**	**4 Rounds of** :15 Jumping Jack :15 Squat :15 MC :15 Jump Squat
EQUIPMENT	BB 225/155 BB 135/95	BB: 155/105	
WOD	DL OHS **21, 15, 9 for time**	**5 Rounds of** FSQ: 7 T2B: 10	Lunge: 25yds (25/15 plate held overhead) Run: 50 **AMRAP: 12 Minutes**
LIFTING/SKILL	CL: 1 every :30 **for 10 Minutes** @80% of 1RM	*Organized Mobility*	Burpee: 10 Wall Ball:10 (Dynamax 20/14) **AMRAP: 10 Minutes**
GAMES Phase II	All	**Active Rest+Games WOD+PH**	All
SKILL/DEV WORK	HSPU: 5 (To AbMat from plates) American Swing: 12 **3 Rounds for time**	Run: 5k (Recover & Stretch) Ankles up	Run: 400 x 6 - **Rest 1:00** Hand Walk: 40ft **Note: Sub wall walk: if no hand walk (15)** KB FSQ 12-12-12-12-12 **EMOTM** (24kg/16kg) Pull Up: 20 (w/#20 Vest)
GAMES WOD	PSN: 2 every :15 x 16 Intervals (135/95)	Thruster: 10 **EMOTM for 10 Minutes** (135/95)	Burpee: 10 Double Under: 30 **3 Rounds for time**
ACCESSORY	GHD Hip/Back Ext: 10 GHD Sit Up: 10 **3 Rounds (Completion)**		Swing: 15-15-15-15-15 **EMOTM** #124/#88
POWER HOUR		Pull Up: 3 Dip: 3 PU - Wide Grip: 3 Dip: 3 PU - Narrow: 3 Dip: 3 PU - Reverse: 3 Dip: 3 PU - MC/R: 3 Dip: 3 PU - MC/L: 3 Dip: 3 **All Movements Strict**	**5 Rounds of** MU Transition: 3 HSPU: 3 (to paralletes) - **Scale on a box, ROM trumps loading**

WEDNESDAY 4/11	THURSDAY 4/12	FRIDAY 4/13	SATURDAY 4/14
4 Rounds of :15 Jumping Jack :15 Squat :15 MC :15 Jump Squat	Run: 400 30/20/30 **Mobility: 10 Minutes**	Run: 400 30/20/30 **Mobility: 10 Minutes**	**4 Rounds of** :15 Jumping Jack :15 Squat :15 MC :15 Jump Squat
	DB 35/25 Slammer: 30/20	Butcher 90/50 DB: 35/25	KB 24/16
Run: 200 Burpee: 10 **AMRAP: 22 Minutes**	**A1** : Run 50yds **A2** : Push Press (Score) **A3** : Ball Slam (Score) **AMRAP: 12 Minutes**	**A1** : Butcher HiPush: 50yds **A2** : Thruster (Score) **A3** Push Up (HR) (Score) **AMRAP: 12 Minutes**	*Helen*
Organized Mobility	*Organized Mobility*	*Organized Mobility*	*Organized Mobility*
All	**Active Rest+PH**	**Games Only**	**All**
MU Transition: 10 DHPU: 10 Dip: 10 Ring Dips: 10 Ring Row (Strict): 1 MU (Strict): 10 HSPU: 10 L-Sit - :20/:10 x 8 Rope Climbs: 5	Run: 5k (Recover & Stretch) Ankles up	Thruster: 3 (155/105) DL: 6 (315/205) **5 Rounds for time**	Sled Drag: 1 Mile (135/90) **for time**
		Butcher HiPush: 50yds (180/120) Burpee: 10 **AMRAP: 20 Minutes**	MU: 30 **for time**
Olympic Lifting		CL&J - **Prison Rules** - 2 Reps every :15 x 16 (135/95)	*Olympic Lifting*
3 Rounds of Rope Climb: 1 BSQ: 12 (225/155)	PJ: 1-1-1-1-1-1-1 EMOTM @1RM		

243

WEEK 37 - SUN APR 08 2012

PHASE II:
Games Track Athletes - All

WARMUP:
With empty bar
3 Rounds of
DL: 3
PCL: 3
FSQ: 3
PJ: 3
OHS: 3

EQUIPMENT:
BB 225/155; BB 135/95

WOD:
DL
OHS
21, 15, 9 for time

LIFTING/SKILL DEV:
CL: 1 every :30 for 10 Minutes
(80% of 1RM)

SKILL/DEV. WORK:
HSPU: 5 (To AbMat from plates)
American Swing: 12
3 Rounds for time

GAMES WOD:
PSN: 2 every :15 x 16 Intervals
(135/95)

ACCESSORY:
GHD Hip/Back Ext: 10
GHD Sit Up: 10
3 Rounds - Completion

WEEK 37 - MON APR 09 2012

PHASE II:
Games Track Athletes -
Active Rest + Games WOD
+ Power Hour

WARMUP:
Run: 400
30/20/30
Mobility: 10 Minutes

EQUIPMENT: BB: 155/105
WOD:
5 Rounds of
FSQ: 7
T2B: 10

LIFTING/SKILL DEV:
Organized Mobility

SKILL/DEV.
NOTE: INSTEAD OF CLASS
Run: 5k (Recover & Stretch)
Ankles up

GAMES WOD:
Thruster: 10 EMOTM
for 10 Minutes (135/95)

POWER HOUR:
NOTE: INSTEAD OF CLASS
Pull Up: 3
Dip: 3
PU - Wide Grip: 3
Dip: 3
PU - Narrow: 3
Dip: 3
PU - Reverse: 3
Dip: 3
PU - Mountain Climber: 3
Dip: 3
PU - Mountain Climber: 3
Dip: 3
All Movements Strict

WEEK 37 -
TUE APR 10 2012

PHASE II:
Games Track Athletes - All

WARMUP:
4 Rounds of
:15 Jumping Jack
:15 Squat
:15 Mountain Climber
:15 Jump Squat

WOD:
Lunge: 25yds
(25/15 plate held overhead)
Run: 50yds
AMRAP: 12 Minutes

LIFTING/SKILL DEV:
Burpee: 10
Wall Ball: 10 (Dynamax 20/14)
AMRAP: 10 Minutes

SKILL/DEV. WORK:
NOTE: INSTEAD OF CLASS
Run: 400 x 6 - 1:00 Rest
Hand Walk: 40ft
Note: Sub wall walk:
if no hand walk (15)
KB FSQ: 12-12-12-12-12
EMOTM (24kg/16kg)
Pull Up: 20 (w/#20 Vest)

GAMES WOD:
NOTE: IN ADDITION TO CLASS
Burpee: 10
Double Under: 30
3 Rounds for time

ACCESSORY:
NOTE: IN ADDITION TO CLASS
Swing: 15-15-15-15-15 EMOTM
(#124/#88)

POWER HOUR:
NOTE: IN ADDITION TO CLASS
5 Rounds of
MU Transitions: 3
HSPU: 3 (to parallets) -
Scale on a box -
ROM trumps loading

WEEK 37 -
WED APR 11 2012

PHASE II:
Games Track Athletes - All

WARMUP:
4 Rounds of
:15 Jumping Jack
:15 Squat
:15 Mountain Climber
:15 Jump Squat

WOD:
Run: 200
Burpee: 10
AMRAP: 22 Minutes

LIFTING/SKILL DEV:
Organized Mobility

SKILL/DEV. WORK:
NOTE: IN ADDITION TO CLASS
MU Transitions: 10
DHPU: 10
Dip: 10
Ring Dips: 10
Ring Row: 10 (Strict)
MU: 10 (Strict)
HSPU: 10
L-Sit - :20/:10 x 8
Rope Climbs: 5

ACCESSORY:
NOTE: IN ADDITION TO CLASS
Olympic Lifting

POWER HOUR:
NOTE: IN ADDITION TO CLASS
3 Rounds of
Rope Climb: 1
BSQ: 12 (225/155)

245

WEEK 37 - THU APR 12 2012

PHASE II:
Games Track Athletes -
Active Rest + Power Hour

WARMUP:
Run: 400
30/20/30
Mobility: 10 Minutes

EQUIPMENT:
DB 35/25; Slammer: 30/20

WOD:
P1: Run 50yds
P2: Push Press (Score)
P3: Ball Slam (Score)

LIFTING/SKILL DEV:
Organized Mobility

SKILL/DEV. WORK:
Run: 5k (Recover & Stretch)
Ankles up

POWER HOUR:
PJ: 1-1-1-1-1-1-1

WEEK 37 - FRI APR 13 2012

PHASE II:
Games Track Athletes -
Games Track

WARMUP:
Run: 400
30/20/30
Mobility: 10 Minutes

EQUIPMENT:
Butcher 90/50; DB: 35/25

WOD:
P1: Butcher Hi Push: 50yds
P2: Thruster (Score)
P3: Push Up: HR (Score)

LIFTING/SKILL DEV:
Organized Mobility

SKILL/DEV. WORK:
NOTE: INSTEAD OF CLASS
Thruster: 3 (155/105)
DL: 6 (315/205)
5 Rounds for time

GAMES WOD:
NOTE: INSTEAD OF CLASS
Butcher Hi Push: 50yds (180/120)
Burpee: 10
AMRAP: 20 Minutes

ACCESSORY:
NOTE: INSTEAD OF CLASS
CL&J - Prison Rules - 2 Reps
every :15 x 16 (135/95)

WEEK 37 -
SAT APR 14 2012

PHASE II:
Games Track Athletes - All

WARMUP:
4 Rounds of
:15 Jumping Jack
:15 Squat
:15 Mountain Climber
:15 Jump Squat

EQUIPMENT: KB 24/16

WOD:
Helen

LIFTING/SKILL DEV:
Organized Mobility

SKILL/DEV. WORK:
NOTE: IN ADDITION TO CLASS
Sled Drag: 1 Mile
(135/90) for time

GAMES WOD:
NOTE: IN ADDITION TO CLASS
Muscle Up: 30 for time

ACCESSORY:
NOTE: IN ADDITION TO CLASS
Olympic Lifting

Week 38

	SUNDAY 4/15	MONDAY 4/16	TUESDAY 4/17
WARM UP	**4 Rounds of** :15 Jumping Jack :15 Squat :15 MC :15 Jump Squat	Run: 400 30/20/30	**4 Rounds of** :15 Jumping Jack :15 Squat :15 MC :15 Jump Squat
EQUIPMENT			BB 125/80
W O D	*Kelly*	Run: 200 Air Squat: 30 **5 Rounds for time**	PJ: 12 Burpee: 10 **5 Rounds for time**
LIFTING/SKILL		*Organized Warmdown*	*Organized Warmdown*
GAMES **Phase II**	All	**Skill/Dev+Games** **WOD+PH**	All
SKILL/DEV **WORK**	FSQ: 5 (185/125) Pull Up: 7 DL: 12 (185/125) **4 Rounds for time**	Run: 5k (Recover & Stretch) Ankles up	Run: 400 x 6 - **Rest 1:00** Hand Walk: 40ft **Note: Sub wall walk: if no** **hand walk (15)** KB FSQ 12-12-12-12-12 **EMOTM** (24kg/16kg) Pull Up: 20 (w/#20 Vest)
GAMES **W O D**	PSN: 2 every :15 x 16 Intervals (135/95)	Hand Walk: 25yds Air Squat: 50 **5 Rounds for time**	DL: 7 (315/205) Pistol 1R/1L x 10 Double Under: 30 **3 Rounds for time**
ACCESSORY	GHD Hip/Back Ext: 10 GHD Sit Up: 10 **3 Rounds (completion)**		Swing: 15-15-15-15-15 **EMOTM** #124/#88
POWER HOUR		Pull Up: 4 Dip: 4 PU - Wide Grip: 4 Dip: 4 PU - Narrow: 4 Dip: 4 PU - Reverse: 4 Dip: 4 PU - MC/R: 4 Dip: 4 PU - MC/L: 4 Dip: 4 **All Movements Strict**	*Tabata* Holds - Hold :20 - **Transition :10 -** **Alternating Exercises** Ring Support Dip Bottom

WEDNESDAY 4/18	THURSDAY 4/19	FRIDAY 4/20	SATURDAY 4/21
4 Rounds of :15 Jumping Jack :15 Squat :15 MC :15 Jump Squat	Run: 400 30/20/30	Run: 400 30/20/30	**4 Rounds of** :15 Jumping Jack :15 Squat :15 MC :15 Jump Squat
BB: 185/125	KB 32/24	BB: 155/105	
PCL 7 T2B: 10 Double Under: 30 **5 Rounds for time**	**A1**: Run 100 **A2**: Push Up (Score) **A3**: Swing (Score) **AMRAP: 12 Minutes**	OHS: 5 Dip: 10 **4 Rounds for time**	*Diane*
Organized Warmdown	*Organized Warmdown*	*Organized Warmdown*	*Organized Warmdown*
All	**Skill/Dev+PH**	**Games Only**	**All**
MU Transition: 10 DHPU: 10 Dip: 10 Ring Dips: 10 Ring Row (Strict): 10 MU (Strict): 10 HSPU: 10 L-Sit - :20/:10 x 8 Rope Climbs: 5	Row: 5k (Recover & Stretch) Ankles up	FSQ: 7 (225/155) Row: 250 Handle Carry: 60ft (90/70) **3 Rounds for time**	
		Butcher LoPush: 25yds (70/50) Run: 50yds **EMOTM for 12 Minutes**	Muscle Up CL&J (225/155) **5, 4, 3, 2, 1 for time**
Olympic Lifting		CL&J - **Prison Rules** - 2 Reps every :15 x 16 (135/95)	*Olympic Lifting*
Thruster: 2 every :15 for 16 intervals (#135/95)	Spring: 100 Jog 100 **AMRAP: 15 Minutes**		

WEEK 38 -
SUN APR 15 2012

PHASE II:
Games Track Athletes - All

WARMUP:
4 Rounds of
:15 Jumping Jack
:15 Squat
:15 Mountain Climber
:15 Jump Squat

WOD:
Kelly

SKILL/DEV. WORK:
NOTE: IN ADDITION TO CLASS
FSQ: 5 (185/125)
Pull Up: 7
DL: 12 (185/125)
4 Rounds for time

GAMES WOD:
NOTE: IN ADDITION TO CLASS
PSN: 2 every :15 x 16 Intervals
(135/95)

ACCESSORY:
NOTE: IN ADDITION TO CLASS
GHD Hip/Back Ext: 10
GHD Sit Up: 10
3 Rounds - Completion

WEEK 38 -
MON APR 16 2012

PHASE II:
Games Track Athletes -
Active Rest + Power Hours

WARMUP:
Run: 400
30/20/30
WOD:
Run: 200
Air Squat: 30
5 Rounds for time

LIFTING/SKILL DEV:
Organized Warmdown

SKILL/DEV. WORK:
NOTE: IN ADDITION TO CLASS
Run: 5k (Recover & Stretch)
Ankles up

GAMES WOD:
NOTE: IN ADDITION TO CLASS
Hand Walk: 25yds
Air Squat: 50
5 Rounds for time

POWER HOUR:
NOTE: IN ADDITION TO CLASS
Pull Up: 4
Dip: 4
PU - Wide Grip: 4
Dip: 4
PU - Narrow: 4
Dip: 4
PU - Reverse: 4
Dip: 4
PU - Mountain Climber: 4
Dip: 4
PU - Mountain Climber: 4
Dip: 4
All Movements Strict

WEEK 38 -
TUE APR 17 2012

PHASE II:
Games Track Athletes - All

WARMUP:
4 Rounds of
:15 Jumping Jack
:15 Squat
:15 Mountain Climber
:15 Jump Squat

EQUIPMENT: BB 125/80

WOD:
PJ: 12
Burpee: 10
5 Rounds for time

LIFTING/SKILL DEV:
Organized Warmdown

SKILL/DEV. WORK:
NOTE: IN ADDITION TO CLASS
Run: 400 x 6 - 1:00 Rest
Hand Walk: 40ft
Note: Sub wall walk:
if no hand walk (15)
KB FSQ: 12-12-12-12-12
EMOTM (24kg/16kg)
Pull Up: 20 (w/#20 Vest)

GAMES WOD:
NOTE: IN ADDITION TO CLASS
DL: 7 (315/205)
Pistol: 1R/1L x 10
Double Under: 30
3 Rounds for time

ACCESSORY:
NOTE: IN ADDITION TO CLASS
Swing: 15-15-15-15-15
EMOTM (#124/#88)

POWER HOUR:
NOTE: IN ADDITION TO CLASS
Tabata Holds
Alternating Exercises
Ring Support
Dip Bottom
:20 Hold - :10 Transition

WEEK 38 -
WED APR 18 2012

PHASE II:
Games Track Athletes - All

WARMUP:
4 Rounds of
:15 Jumping Jack
:15 Squat
:15 Mountain Climber
:15 Jump Squat

EQUIPMENT: BB: 185/125

WOD:
PCL: 7
T2B: 10
Double Under: 30
5 Rounds for time

LIFTING/SKILL DEV:
Organized Warmdown

SKILL/DEV. WORK:
NOTE: IN ADDITION TO CLASS
MU Transitions: 10
DHPU: 10
Dip: 10
Ring Dips: 10
Ring Row (Strict): 10
MU (Strict): 10
HSPU: 10
L-Sit - :20/:10 x 8
Rope Climbs: 5

ACCESSORY:
NOTE: IN ADDITION TO CLASS
Olympic Lifting

POWER HOUR:
NOTE: IN ADDITION TO CLASS
Thruster: 2 every :15 for 16
intervals (#135/95)

251

WEEK 38 - THU APR 19 2012

PHASE II:
Games Track Athletes -
Active Rest

WARMUP:
Run: 400
30/20/30

EQUIPMENT: KB 32/24

WOD:
P1: Run: 100
P2: Push Up (Score)
P3: Swing (Score)

LIFTING/SKILL DEV:
Organized Warmdown

SKILL/DEV. WORK:
NOTE: INSTEAD OF CLASS
Row: 5k (Recover & Stretch)
Ankles up

POWER HOUR:
NOTE: INSTEAD OF CLASS
Sprint: 100 - Jog: 100 -
AMRAP: 15 Minutes

WEEK 38 - FRI APR 20 2012

PHASE II:
Games Track Athletes -
All

WARMUP:
Run: 400
30/20/30

EQUIPMENT:
BB: 155/105

WOD:
OHS: 5
Dip: 10
4 Rounds for time

LIFTING/SKILL DEV:
Organized Warmdown

SKILL/DEV. WORK:
NOTE: INSTEAD OF CLASS
FSQ: 7 (225/155)
Row: 250
Handle Carry: 60ft (90/70)
3 Rounds for time

GAMES WOD:
NOTE: INSTEAD OF CLASS
Low Push: 25yds (70/50)
Run: 50yds
EMOTM for 12 Minutes

ACCESSORY:
NOTE: INSTEAD OF CLASS
CL&J - Prison Rules -
2 Reps every :15 x 16
(135/95)

WEEK 38 -
SAT APR 21 2012

PHASE II:
Games Track Athletes -
All

WARMUP:
4 Rounds of
:15 Jumping Jack
:15 Squat
:15 Mountain Climber
:15 Jump Squat

WOD:
Diane

LIFTING/SKILL DEV:
Organized Warmdown

GAMES WOD:
NOTE: INSTEAD OF CLASS
Muscle Up
CL&J (225/155)
5, 4, 3, 2, 1 for time

ACCESSORY:
NOTE: INSTEAD OF CLASS
Olympic Lifting

Week 39

	SUNDAY 4/22	MONDAY 4/23	TUESDAY 4/24
WARM UP	**4 Rounds of** :15 Jumping Jack :15 Squat :15 Mountain Climber :15 Jump Squat **Then** Run/lunge 2x Run/butt kickers 2x Run/power skips 2x Run/Spidey 2x Run/inchworm 2x **Then 4 Rounds of** :15 Plank :15 Superman :15 Side Plank /L :15 Side Plank /R	**4 Rounds of** :15 Jumping Jack :15 Squat :15 Mountain Climber :15 Jump Squat **Then** Run/lunge 2x Run/butt kickers 2x Run/power skips 2x Run/Spidey 2x Run/inchworm 2x **Then 4 Rounds of** :15 Plank :15 Superman :15 Side Plank /L :15 Side Plank /R	**4 Rounds of** :15 Jumping Jack :15 Squat :15 Mountain Climber :15 Jump Squat **Then** Run/lunge 2x Run/butt kickers 2x Run/power skips 2x Run/Spidey 2x Run/inchworm 2x **Then 4 Rounds of** :15 Plank :15 Superman :15 Side Plank /L :15 Side Plank /R
EQUIPMENT	BB 135/95	Butcher 70/50	Jump Rope
WOD	SN: 4 CL&J:6 (ground to overhead) DL: 9 **7 Rounds for time**	**A1**: Butcher HiPush: 25yds **A2**: Butcher LoPush: 25yds **A3**: Butcher HiPush: 25yds **AMRAP: 15 Minutes**	*Annie*
LIFTING/SKILL		*Active Warm Down*	*Active Warm Down*
GAMES Phase II	All	Skill/Dev+Games WOD+PH	All
SKILL/DEV WORK	DB High Pull 1/1 x 10 (#70) DB SN: 1/1 x 5 HSPU: 10 **(anyhow)** **Then** Waiter's Walk /R: 25yds #50 Burpees: 10 Waiter's Walk /L: 25yds #50 Burpees: 10 **AMRAP: 5 Minutes**	Do WARMUP Row: 2,000M (90% Pace) Ankles Up	DB High Pull 1/1 x 10 (#70) DB SN: 1/1 x 5 HSPU: 10 **(anyhow)** **Then** Waiter's Walk /R: 25yds #50 Burpees: 10 Waiter's Walk /L: 25yds #50 Burpees: 10 **AMRAP: 5 Minutes** Pistol: 1R/1L x 10
GAMES WOD	Row: 2k Pistol: 1R/1L 50 HCL: 30 (225/135) **For time**	**Work on specific regional needs for you. i.e. work on the things that challenge you.**	Double Under: 20 SN: 1 (125) **Every :45 for 12 Intervals**
ACCESSORY	Swing: 10 124/88 DU: 15 **EMOTM for 5 Minutes**		BSQ: 2-2-2-2-2-2-2-2-2-2 **EMOTM @90% of 1RM**
POWER HOUR		SN Grip DL from Plates: 3 every :20 for 12 intervals - 225/155	HCL&J - **Prison Rules** - (All from hang) R12.2 Standard - 155/105

WEDNESDAY 4/25	THURSDAY 4/26	FRIDAY 4/27	SATURDAY 4/28
4 Rounds of :15 Jumping Jack :15 Squat :15 Mountain Climber :15 Jump Squat **Then** Run/lunge 2x Run/butt kickers 2x Run/power skips 2x Run/Spidey 2x Run/inchworm 2x **Then 4 Rounds of** :15 Plank :15 Superman :15 Side Plank /L :15 Side Plank /R	**4 Rounds of** :15 Jumping Jack :15 Squat :15 Mountain Climber :15 Jump Squat **Then** Run/lunge 2x Run/butt kickers 2x Run/power skips 2x Run/Spidey 2x Run/inchworm 2x **Then 4 Rounds of** :15 Plank :15 Superman :15 Side Plank /L :15 Side Plank /R	**4 Rounds of** :15 Jumping Jack :15 Squat :15 Mountain Climber :15 Jump Squat **Then** Run/lunge 2x Run/butt kickers 2x Run/power skips 2x Run/Spidey 2x Run/inchworm 2x **Then 4 Rounds of** :15 Plank :15 Superman :15 Side Plank /L :15 Side Plank /R	**4 Rounds of** :15 Jumping Jack :15 Squat :15 Mountain Climber :15 Jump Squat **Then** Run/lunge 2x Run/butt kickers 2x Run/power skips 2x Run/Spidey 2x Run/inchworm 2x **Then 4 Rounds of** :15 Plank :15 Superman :15 Side Plank /L :15 Side Plank /R
Dynamax 20/14 Slammer 30/20	DB 35/25		BB 95/65
Wall Ball: 7 Ball Slam: 7 Run: 100 **AMRAP: 5 Minutes -** **Rest 1:00 - 5 Rounds**	Run: 200 T2B: 12 Thruster: 12 **AMRAP: 17 Minutes**	Run: 800 **Then 10 Rounds of** *Cindy* for time	*Coe*
		Active Warm Down	*Active Warm Down*
All+ O-Lifting	**Skill/Dev Only**	**All**	**All**
5 Rounds of Pull Up: 10 (#20 Vest) Dip*: 10 (#20 Vest) **Then 5 Rounds** Pull Up: 10 Dip*: 10 *Kip or anyhow	Row: 5k Ankles Up	**3 Rounds of** DL: 7 (345/225) MU: 7 **Then 3 Rounds of** Wall Ball: 21 T2B: 21 **Then** Farmer's Walk: 100ft Burpee Box Jumps: 28 Farmer's Walk: 100ft Muscle Up: 3 **For time**	DB High Pull 1/1 x 10 (#70) DB SN: 1/1 x 5 HSPU: 10 **(anyhow)** **Then** Waiter's Walk /R: 25yds #50 Burpees: 10 Waiter's Walk /L: 25yds #50 Burpees: 10 **AMRAP: 5 Minutes**
DL: 2 every :15 for 16 Intervals - (315/205)		**30 Minutes between WOD** **and DL**	Run: 200 FSQ: Max Reps (185/125) **AMRAP: 15 Minutes -** **Track total FSQ**
OHS 2-2-2-2-2-2-2-2-2-2 **EMOTM** @90%of 1RM		DL: 2-2-2-2-2-2-2-2-2-2 **EMOTM** @90%of 1RM	Swing: 10 - 124/88 DU: 15 **EMOTM for 5 Minutes**
SN Grip DL from Plates: 3 every :20 for 12 intervals - 225/155			

WEEK 39 - SUN APR 22 2012

PHASE II:
Games Track Athletes - All

WARMUP:
4 Rounds of
:15 Jumping Jack
:15 Squat
:15 Mountain Climber
:15 Jump Squat
Then
Run/lunge 2x
Run/butt kickers 2x
Run/power skips 2x
Run/Spidey 2x
Run/inchworm 2x
Then 4 Rounds of
:15 Plank
:15 Superman
:15 Side Plank - L
:15 Side Plank - R

EQUIPMENT: BB 135/95

WOD:
SN: 4
CL&J: 6 (ground to overhead)
DL: 9
7 Rounds for time

SKILL/DEV. WORK:
NOTE: IN ADDITION TO CLASS
DB High Pull: 1/1 x 10 (#70)
DB SN: 1/1 x 5
HSPU: 10 (anyhow)
Then
Waiter's Walk: 25yds (R) #50
Burpees: 10
Waiter's Walk: 25yds (L) #50
Burpees: 10
AMRAP: 5 Minutes

GAMES WOD:
NOTE: IN ADDITION TO CLASS
Row: 2k
Pistol: 1R/1L x 50
HCL: 30 (225/135)
For time

ACCESSORY:
NOTE: IN ADDITION TO CLASS
Swing: 10 (124/88)
DU: 15
EMOTM for 5 Minutes

WEEK 39 - MON APR 23 2012

PHASE II:
Games Track Athletes -
Active Rest + Power Hour

WARMUP:
4 Rounds of
:15 Jumping Jack
:15 Squat
:15 Mountain Climber
:15 Jump Squat
Then
Run/lunge 2x
Run/butt kickers 2x
Run/power skips 2x
Run/Spidey 2x
Run/inchworm 2x
Then 4 Rounds of
:15 Plank
:15 Superman
:15 Side Plank - L
:15 Side Plank - R

EQUIPMENT: Butcher 70/50

WOD:
P1: High Push: 25yds
P2: Low Push: 25yds
P3: High Push 25yds
AMRAP: 15 Minutes

CONTINUED>>>>>>

LIFTING/SKILL DEV:
Active Warm Down

SKILL/DEV. WORK:
NOTE: INSTEAD OF CLASS
Do Class WARMUP
Row: 2,000M (90% Pace)
Ankles Up

GAMES WOD:
NOTE: INSTEAD OF CLASS
Work on specific regional needs
for you; i.e. work on the things
that challenge you.

POWER HOUR:
NOTE: INSTEAD OF CLASS
SN Grip DL from Plates:
3 every :20 for 12 intervals
(225/155)

WEEK 39 -
TUE APR 24 2012

PHASE II:
Games Track Athletes - All

WARMUP:
4 Rounds of
:15 Jumping Jack
:15 Squat
:15 Mountain Climber
:15 Jump Squat
Then
Run/lunge 2x
Run/butt kickers 2x
Run/power skips 2x
Run/Spidey 2x
Run/inchworm 2x
Then 4 Rounds of
:15 Plank
:15 Superman
:15 Side Plank - L
:15 Side Plank - R

EQUIPMENT:
Jump Rope

WOD:
Annie

LIFTING/SKILL DEV:
Active Warm Down

SKILL/DEV. WORK:
NOTE: IN ADDITION TO CLASS
DB High Pull 1/1 x 10 (#70)
DB SN: 1/1 x 5
HSPU: 10 (anyhow)
Then
Waiter's Walk: 25yds (R) #50
Burpees: 10
Waiter's Walk: 25yds (L) #50
Burpees: 10
AMRAP: 5 Minutes
Then
Pistol: 1R/1L x 10

GAMES WOD:
NOTE: IN ADDITION TO CLASS
Double Under: 20
SN: 1 (125)
Every :45 for 12 Intervals

ACCESSORY:
NOTE: IN ADDITION TO CLASS
BSQ: 2-2-2-2-2-2-2-2-2-2 EMOTM

POWER HOUR:
NOTE: IN ADDITION TO CLASS
HCL&J - Prison Rules
(All from hang) -
R12.2 Standard (155/105)

WEEK 39 -
WED APR 25 2012

PHASE II:
Games Track Athletes - All

WARMUP:
4 Rounds of
:15 Jumping Jack
:15 Squat
:15 Mountain Climber
:15 Jump Squat
Then
Run/lunge 2x
Run/butt kickers 2x
Run/power skips 2x
Run/Spidey 2x
Run/inchworm 2x
Then 4 Rounds of
:15 Plank
:15 Superman
:15 Side Plank - L
:15 Side Plank - R

EQUIPMENT:
Dynamax 20/14;
Slammer 30/20

WOD:
Wall Ball: 7
Ball Slam: 7
Run: 100
AMRAP: 5 Minutes - Rest 1:00 -
5 Rounds

SKILL/DEV. WORK:
*NOTE: IN ADDITION TO CLASS,
AND FOLLOWED BY O-LIFTING*
Pull Up: 10 (#20 Vest)
Dip: 10 (#20 Vest) - Kip or anyhow
Then 5 Rounds of
Pull Up: 10
Dip: 10 - Kip or anyhow

GAMES WOD:
*NOTE: IN ADDITION TO CLASS,
AND FOLLOWED BY O-LIFTING*
DL: 2 every :15 for 16 Intervals
(315/205)

ACCESSORY:
*NOTE: IN ADDITION TO CLASS,
AND FOLLOWED BY O-LIFTING*
OHS 2-2-2-2-2-2-2-2-2-2 EMOTM

POWER HOUR:
*NOTE: IN ADDITION TO CLASS,
AND FOLLOWED BY O-LIFTING*
SN Grip DL from Plates:
3 every :20 for 12 intervals
(225/155)

WEEK 39 -
THU APR 26 2012

PHASE II:
Games Track Athletes -
Active Rest
WARMUP:
4 Rounds of
:15 Jumping Jack
:15 Squat
:15 Mountain Climber
:15 Jump Squat
Then
Run/lunge 2x
Run/butt kickers 2x
Run/power skips 2x
Run/Spidey 2x
Run/inchworm 2x
Then 4 Rounds of
:15 Plank
:15 Superman
:15 Side Plank - L
:15 Side Plank - R
WOD:
Run: 200
T2B: 12
Thruster: 12
AMRAP: 17 Minutes
SKILL/DEV. WORK:
NOTE: INSTEAD OF CLASS
Row: 5k
Ankles Up

WEEK 39 - FRI APR 27 2012

PHASE II:
Games Track Athletes - All

WARMUP:
4 Rounds of
:15 Jumping Jack
:15 Squat
:15 Mountain Climber
:15 Jump Squat
Then
Run/lunge 2x
Run/butt kickers 2x
Run/power skips 2x
Run/Spidey 2x
Run/inchworm 2x
Then 4 Rounds of
:15 Plank
:15 Superman
:15 Side Plank - L
:15 Side Plank - R

EQUIPMENT: DB 35/25

WOD:
Run: 800
Then 10 Rounds of Cindy
For time

LIFTING/SKILL DEV:
Active Warm Down

SKILL/DEV. WORK:
NOTE: IN ADDITION TO CLASS
3 Rounds of
DL: 7 (345/225)
MU: 7
Then 3 Rounds of
Wall Ball: 21
T2B: 21
Then
Farmer's Walk: 100ft
Burpee Box Jump: 28
Farmer's Walk: 100ft
Muscle Up: 3
For time

GAMES WOD:
NOTE: IN ADDITION TO CLASS
30 Minutes between WOD and DL

ACCESSORY:
NOTE: IN ADDITION TO CLASS
DL: 2-2-2-2-2-2-2-2-2-2 EMOTM!

WEEK 39 - SAT APR 28 2012

PHASE II:
Games Track Athletes - All

WARMUP:
4 Rounds of
:15 Jumping Jack
:15 Squat
:15 Mountain Climber
:15 Jump Squat
Then
Run/lunge 2x
Run/butt kickers 2x
Run/power skips 2x
Run/Spidey 2x
Run/inchworm 2x
Then 4 Rounds of
:15 Plank
:15 Superman
:15 Side Plank - L
:15 Side Plank - R

EQUIPMENT: BB 95/65

WOD:
Coe

LIFTING/SKILL DEV:
Active Warm Down

SKILL/DEV. WORK:
NOTE: IN ADDITION TO CLASS
DB High Pull: 1/1 x 10 (#70)
DB SN: 1/1 x 5
HSPU: 10 (anyhow)
Then
Waiter's Walk: 25yds (R) #50
Burpees: 10
Waiter's Walk: 25yds (L) #50
Burpees: 10
AMRAP: 5 Minutes

GAMES WOD:
NOTE: IN ADDITION TO CLASS
Run: 200
FSQ: Max Reps (185/125)
AMRAP: 15 Minutes -
Track total FSQ

ACCESSORY:
NOTE: IN ADDITION TO CLASS
Swing: 10 (124/88)
DU: 15
EMOTM for 5 Minutes

259

Week 40

	SUNDAY 4/29	MONDAY 4/30	TUESDAY 5/1
WARM UP	**4 Rounds of** :15 Jumping Jack :15 Squat :15 Mountain Climber :15 Jump Squat	**4 Rounds of** :15 Jumping Jack :15 Squat :15 Mountain Climber :15 Jump Squat **Then** Run/lunge 2x Run/butt kickers 2x Run/Straight Leg March 2x Run/power skips 2x Run/Spidey 2x Run/inchworm 2x **Then 4 Rounds of** :15 Plank :15 Superman :15 Side Plank /L :15 Side Plank /R	**4 Rounds of** :15 Jumping Jack :15 Squat :15 Mountain Climber :15 Jump Squat **Then** Run/lunge 2x Run/butt kickers 2x Run/Straight Leg March 2x Run/power skips 2x Run/Spidey 2x Run/inchworm 2x **Then 4 Rounds of** :15 Plank :15 Superman :15 Side Plank /L :15 Side Plank /R
EQUIPMENT	BB (Regional Loading)		DB: 35/24
W O D	BSQ: 50 (135/95) Pull Up: 40 Push Press: 30 (135/95) FSQ: 50 (85/65) Pull Up: 40 Push Press: 30 (85/65) OHS: 50 (65/45) Pull Up: 40 Push Press: 30 (65/45) **For time**	**A1**: Run: 100 **A2**: Wall Ball (Score) **A3**: Burpee **AMRAP: 12 Minutes**	Run: 100 Thruster: 7 Pull Up: 7 **AMRAP: 7 Minutes - Rest 3:00 - 2 Rounds**
GAMES Phase II	All	Skill/Dev+PH	All
SKILL/DEV WORK	DB High Pull 1/1 x 10 (#70) DB SN: 1/1 x 5 HSPU: 10 **(anyhow)** **Then** Waiter's Walk /R: 25yds #50 Burpees: 10 Waiter's Walk /L: 25yds #50 Burpees: 10 **AMRAP: 5 Minutes** Pistols: 1R/1L x 10	Row 2k (90% of Max Rate) Ankles Up	HSPU: 5 **EMOTM for 10 Minutes**
GAMES W O D	3 Rounds of Pistols: 1R/1L x 10 Double Under: 20 Deadlift: 5 (345/225)		ButcherHiPush:25yds(70/50) ButcherLoPush:25yds(70/50) Run: 100 **AMRAP: 12 Minutes**
ACCESSORY	Sled Drag: 800 (135/90)		GHD Sit Up: 12 Swing: 12 (88/124) **5 Rounds for time**
POWER HOUR		Block Cleans (High Position): 15 (225/135)	BSQ: 2-2-2-2-2-2-2-2-2 **EMOTM**

WEDNESDAY 5/2	THURSDAY 5/3	FRIDAY 5/4	SATURDAY 5/5
4 Rounds of :15 Jumping Jack :15 Squat :15 Mountain Climber :15 Jump Squat **Then** Run/lunge 2x Run/butt kickers 2x Run/Straight Leg March 2x Run/power skips 2x Run/Spidey 2x Run/inchworm 2x **Then 4 Rounds of** :15 Plank :15 Superman :15 Side Plank /L :15 Side Plank /R	**4 Rounds of** :15 Jumping Jack :15 Squat :15 Mountain Climber :15 Jump Squat **Then** Run/lunge 2x Run/butt kickers 2x Run/Straight Leg March 2x Run/power skips 2x Run/Spidey 2x Run/inchworm 2x **Then 4 Rounds of** :15 Plank :15 Superman :15 Side Plank /L :15 Side Plank /R	**4 Rounds of** :15 Jumping Jack :15 Squat :15 Mountain Climber :15 Jump Squat **Then** Run/lunge 2x Run/butt kickers 2x Run/Straight Leg March 2x Run/power skips 2x Run/Spidey 2x Run/inchworm 2x **Then 4 Rounds of** :15 Plank :15 Superman :15 Side Plank /L :15 Side Plank /R	**4 Rounds of** :15 Jumping Jack :15 Squat :15 Mountain Climber :15 Jump Squat
	KB 24/16 AbMat	Butcher #70/50	
Run: 200 Lunge 25yds Broad Jump 25yds **5 Rounds for time**	Swing: 21 Push Up: 21 AbMat Sit Up: 21 **5 Rounds for time**	**A1**: Butcher HiPush: 25yds **A2**: Butcher LoPush: 25yds **A3**: Butcher HiPush: 25yds **Cycle Rounds - AMRAP: 4 Minutes - Rest 1:00 - 4 Rounds**	*Roy*

All	Skill/Dev+PH	Games Only	All
3 Rounds of Pull Up: 20 - #20 Vest Dips: 20 - #20 Vest	Row 2k (90% of Max Rate) Ankles Up	**3 Rounds of** Hand Walk 40ft Pull Up: 20 - #20 Vest Dips: 20 - #20 Vest	DB High Pull 1/1 x 10 (#70) DB SN: 1/1 x 5 HSPU: 10 **(anyhow)** **Then** Waiter's Walk /R: 25yds #50 Burpees: 10 Waiter's Walk /L: 25yds #50 Burpees: 10 **AMRAP: 5 Minutes** Pistols: 1R/1L x 10
4 Rounds of DB SN: 5/5 (#100/70) Sprint: 50 Yards		Burpee: 5 SN: 1 (Work up from #85 by #5) **EMOTM until failure**	**7 Rounds of** FSQ: 7 (185/125) Pull Up C2B: 7
Pistols: 1R/1L x 25			
SN Grip DL from Plates: 3 every :20 for 12 intervals - 225/155	DL: 2-2-2-2-2-2-2-2-2 **EMOTM**		

WEEK 40 -
SUN APR 29 2012

PHASE II:
Games Track Athletes - All

WARMUP:
4 Rounds of
:15 Jumping Jack
:15 Squat
:15 Mountain Climber
:15 Jump Squat

EQUIPMENT:
BB (Regional Loading)

WOD:
BSQ: 50 (135/95)
Pull Up: 40
Push Press: 30 (135/95)
FSQ: 50 (85/65)
Pull Up: 40
Push Press: 30 (85/65)
OHS: 50 (65/45)
Pull Up: 40
Push Press: 30 (65/45)
For time

SKILL/DEV. WORK:
NOTE: IN ADDITION TO CLASS
DB High Pull 1/1 x 10 (#70)
DB SN: 1/1 x 5
HSPU: 10 (anyhow)
Then
Waiter's Walk: 25yds (R) #50
Burpees: 10
Waiter's Walk: 25yds (L) #50
Burpees: 10
AMRAP: 5 Minutes
Then
Pistol: 1R/1L x 10

GAMES WOD:
NOTE: IN ADDITION TO CLASS
3 Rounds of
Pistol: 1R/1L x 10
Double Under: 20
Deadlift: 5 (345/225)

ACCESSORY:
NOTE: IN ADDITION TO CLASS
Sled Drag: 800 (135/90)

WEEK 40 -
MON APR 30 2012

PHASE II:
Games Track Athletes -
Active Rest + Power Hour

WARMUP:
4 Rounds of
:15 Jumping Jack
:15 Squat
:15 Mountain Climber
:15 Jump Squat
Then
Run/lunge 2x
Run/butt kickers 2x
Run/Straight Leg March 2x
Run/power skips 2x
Run/Spidey 2x
Run/inchworm 2x
Then 4 Rounds of
:15 Plank
:15 Superman
:15 Side Plank - L
:15 Side Plank - R

WOD:
P1: Run: 100
P2: Wall Ball (Score)
P3: Burpee
AMRAP: 12 Minutes

SKILL/DEV. WORK:
NOTE: INSTEAD OF CLASS
Row 2k (90%)
Ankles Up

POWER HOUR:
NOTE: INSTEAD OF CLASS
Block Cleans (High Position):
15 (225/135)

WEEK 40 - TUE MAY 01 2012

PHASE II:
Games Track Athletes - All

WARMUP:
4 Rounds of
:15 Jumping Jack
:15 Squat
:15 Mountain Climber
:15 Jump Squat
Then
Run/lunge 2x
Run/butt kickers 2x
Run/power skips 2x
Run/Spidey 2x
Run/inchworm 2x
Then 4 Rounds of
:15 Plank
:15 Superman
:15 Side Plank - L
:15 Side Plank - R

EQUIPMENT: DB: 35/24

WOD:
Run: 100
Thruster: 7
Pull Up: 7
AMRAP: 7 Minutes - Rest 3:00
 - 2 Rounds

SKILL/DEV. WORK:
NOTE: IN ADDITION TO CLASS
HSPU: 5 EMOTM for 10 Mins

GAMES WOD:
NOTE: IN ADDITION TO CLASS
Butcher Hi-Push: 25yds (70/50)
Butcher Lo-Push: 25yds (70/50)
Run: 100
AMRAP: 12 Minutes

ACCESSORY:
NOTE: IN ADDITION TO CLASS
GHD Sit Up: 12
Swing: 12 (88/124)
5 Rounds for time

POWER HOUR:
NOTE: IN ADDITION TO CLASS
BSQ: 2-2-2-2-2-2-2-2-2 EMOTM

WEEK 40 - WED MAY 02 2012

PHASE II:
Games Track Athletes - All

WARMUP:
4 Rounds of
:15 Jumping Jack
:15 Squat
:15 Mountain Climber
:15 Jump Squat
Then
Run/lunge 2x
Run/butt kickers 2x
Run/Straight Leg March 2x
Run/power skips 2x
Run/Spidey 2x
Run/inchworm 2x
Then 4 Rounds of
:15 Plank
:15 Superman
:15 Side Plank - L
:15 Side Plank - R

WOD:
Run: 200
Lunge: 25yds
Broad Jump: 25yds
5 Rounds for time

SKILL/DEV. WORK:
NOTE: IN ADDITION TO CLASS
3 Rounds of
Pull Up: 20 (w/#20 Vest)
Dips: 20 (w/#20 Vest)

GAMES WOD:
NOTE: IN ADDITION TO CLASS
4 Rounds of
DB SN: 5/5 (#100/70)
Sprint: 50yds

ACCESSORY:
NOTE: IN ADDITION TO CLASS
Pistol: 1R/1L x 25

POWER HOUR:
NOTE: IN ADDITION TO CLASS
SN Grip DL from Plates:
3 every :20 for 12 intervals
(225/155)

WEEK 40 -
THU MAY 03 2012

PHASE II:
Games Track Athletes -
Active Rest

WARMUP:
4 Rounds of
:15 Jumping Jack
:15 Squat
:15 Mountain Climber
:15 Jump Squat
Then
Run/lunge 2x
Run/butt kickers 2x
Run/Straight Leg March 2x
Run/power skips 2x
Run/Spidey 2x
Run/inchworm 2x
Then 4 Rounds of
:15 Plank
:15 Superman
:15 Side Plank - L
:15 Side Plank - R

EQUIPMENT:
KB 24/16; AbMat

WOD:
Swing: 21
Push Up: 21
AbMat Sit Up: 21
5 Rounds for time

SKILL/DEV. WORK:
NOTE: IN ADDITION TO CLASS
Row 2k (90%)
Ankles Up

POWER HOUR:
NOTE: IN ADDITION TO CLASS
DL: 2-2-2-2-2-2-2-2-2 EMOTM

WEEK 40 -
FRI MAY 04 2012

PHASE II:
Games Track Athletes - All

WARMUP:
4 Rounds of
:15 Jumping Jack
:15 Squat
:15 Mountain Climber
:15 Jump Squat
Then
Run/lunge 2x
Run/butt kickers 2x
Run/Straight Leg March 2x
Run/power skips 2x
Run/Spidey 2x
Run/inchworm 2x
Then 4 Rounds of
:15 Plank
:15 Superman
:15 Side Plank - L
:15 Side Plank - R

EQUIPMENT: Butcher #70/50

WOD:
P1: Butcher Hi-Push: 25yds
P2: Butcher Lo-Push: 25yds
P3: Butcher Hi Push: 25yds
Cycle Rounds
AMRAP: 4 Minutes - Rest 1:00 -
4 Rounds

SKILL/DEV. WORK:
NOTE: IN ADDITION TO CLASS
3 Rounds of
Hand Walk: 40ft
Pull Up: 20 (w/#20 Vest)
Dips: 20 (w/#20 Vest)

GAMES WOD:
NOTE: IN ADDITION TO CLASS
Burpee: 5
SN: 1 (Work up from #85 by #5)
EMOTM until failure

264

WEEK 40 -
SAT MAY 05 2012

PHASE II:
Games Track Athletes - All

WARMUP:
4 Rounds of
:15 Jumping Jack
:15 Squat
:15 Mountain Climber
:15 Jump Squat

WOD:
Roy

SKILL/DEV. WORK:
NOTE: IN ADDITION TO CLASS
DB High Pull 1/1 x 10 (#70)
DB SN: 1/1 x 5
HSPU: 10 (anyhow)
Then
Waiter's Walk: 25yds (R) #50
Burpees: 10
Waiter's Walk: 25yds (L) #50
Burpees: 10
AMRAP: 5 Minutes
Pistol: 1R/1L x 10

GAMES WOD:
NOTE: IN ADDITION TO CLASS
7 Rounds of
FSQ: 7 (185/125)
Pull Up C2B: 7

Week 41

	SUNDAY 5/6	MONDAY 5/7	TUESDAY 5/8
WARM UP	**4 Rounds of** :15 Jumping Jack :15 Squat :15 MC :15 Jump Squat **Then 4 Rounds of** :15 Plank :15 Superman :15 Side Plank /L :15 Side Plank /R	**4 Rounds of** :15 Jumping Jack :15 Squat :15 MC :15 Jump Squat **Then** Run/lunge 2x Run/butt kickers 2x Run/Straight Leg March 2x Run/power skips 2x Run/Spidey 2x Run/Toes Hold 2x Run/inchworm 2x **Then 4 Rounds of** :15 Plank :15 Superman :15 Side Plank /L :15 Side Plank /R	**4 Rounds of** :15 Jumping Jack :15 Squat :15 MC :15 Jump Squat **Then** Run/lunge 2x Run/butt kickers 2x Run/Straight Leg March 2x Run/power skips 2x Run/Spidey 2x Run/Toes Hold 2x Run/inchworm 2x **Then 4 Rounds of** :15 Plank :15 Superman :15 Side Plank /L :15 Side Plank /R
EQUIPMENT	Slammer #30/#20 Wall Ball: #20/#14	DB #35/#25 Dynamax #20/#14	KB 24kg/16kg Slammer #30/#20
WOD	Run: 200 Ball Slam: 9 Wall Ball: 9 **AMRAP: 6 Minutes -** **Rest 3:00 - 4** **Rounds**	**2-Partner WOD** Burpee 1-10 x 1 Push Press 2-20 x 2 Pull Up 1-10 x 1 Wall Ball 2-20 x 2 **For time**	Row: 1000 **Then** American Swing Ball Slam **21, 15, 9 for time**
GAMES Phase II	All	PH Only	All
SKILL/DEV WORK	BSQ: 21 (#135/95) MU: 7 **3 Rounds for time**		Pull Up: 15 T2B : 15 **3 Rounds (Completion)**
GAMES WOD	DL: 2 every :15 for 16 Intervals - #345/#225		DB SN 1/1 x 5 Row: 150 **3 Rounds for time**
ACCESSORY	3 Rounds of HSPU: 7 Burpee Box Jump:12		GHD Sit Up: 12 Swing : 12 (#124/88) **3 Rounds for time**
POWER HOUR		BSQ 5-5-5-5-5 **EMOTM** @80% of 1RM	FSQ 5-5-5-5-5 **EMOTM** @80% of 1RM

266

WEDNESDAY 5/9	THURSDAY 5/10	FRIDAY 5/11	SATURDAY 5/12
4 Rounds of	**4 Rounds of**	**4 Rounds of**	**4 Rounds of**
:15 Jumping Jack	:15 Jumping Jack	:15 Jumping Jack	:15 Jumping Jack
:15 Squat	:15 Squat	:15 Squat	:15 Squat
:15 MC	:15 MC	:15 MC	:15 MC
:15 Jump Squat	:15 Jump Squat	:15 Jump Squat	:15 Jump Squat
Then	**Then**	**Then**	**Then 4 Rounds of**
Run/lunge 2x	Run/lunge 2x	Run/lunge 2x	:15 Plank
Run/butt kickers 2x	Run/butt kickers 2x	Run/butt kickers 2x	:15 Superman
Run/Straight Leg March 2x	Run/Straight Leg March 2x	Run/Straight Leg March 2x	:15 Side Plank /L
Run/power skips 2x	Run/power skips 2x	Run/power skips 2x	:15 Side Plank /R
Run/Spidey 2x	Run/Spidey 2x	Run/Spidey 2x	
Run/Toes Hold 2x	Run/Toes Hold 2x	Run/Toes Hold 2x	
Run/inchworm 2x	Run/inchworm 2x	Run/inchworm 2x	
Then 4 Rounds of	**Then 4 Rounds of**	**Then 4 Rounds of**	
:15 Plank	:15 Plank	:15 Plank	
:15 Superman	:15 Superman	:15 Superman	
:15 Side Plank /L	:15 Side Plank /L	:15 Side Plank /L	
:15 Side Plank /R	:15 Side Plank /R	:15 Side Plank /R	
DB #35/#25	Butcher #70/#50	DB #35/25	BB #135/#95
Run: 100	A1 : Butcher HiPush 25yds	Lunge (High Carry): 25yds	*Amanda*
Burpee: 7	A2 : Butcher LoPush 25yds	Push Press: 10	
Thruster: 7	A3 : Butcher HiPush 25yds	Push Up: 10	
AMRAP: 4 Minutes -Rest	**Cycle Through - AMRAP:**	**AMRAP: 7 Minutes - Rest**	
1:00 - 4 Rounds	**12 Minutes**	**3:00 - 2 Rounds**	
All	**Skill/Dev+PH**	**All**	**All**
Pistols: 1R/1L x 15	Row/Roll prep		
Shoulder to Overhead: 15			
FSQ: 15			
3 Rounds for time -			
#135/#95			
PCL (1+1) x 10 **EMOTM**	PSN (1+1) x 10 **EMOTM**		
@90% of 1RM	@90% of 1RM		

WEEK 41 - SUN MAY 06 2012

PHASE II:
Games Track Athletes - All

WARMUP:
4 Rounds of
:15 Jumping Jack
:15 Squat
:15 Mountain Climber
:15 Jump Squat
Then 4 Rounds of
:15 Plank
:15 Superman
:15 Side Plank - L
:15 Side Plank - R

EQUIPMENT:
Slammer #30/#20;
Wall Ball: #20/#14

WOD:
Run: 200
Ball Slam: 9
Wall Ball: 9
AMRAP: 6 Minutes - Rest 3:00 -
4 Rounds

SKILL/DEV. WORK:
NOTE: IN ADDITION TO CLASS
BSQ: 21 (#135/95)
MU: 7
3 Rounds for time

GAMES WOD:
NOTE: IN ADDITION TO CLASS
DL: 2 every :15 for 16 Intervals -
#345/#225

ACCESSORY:
NOTE: IN ADDITION TO CLASS
3 Rounds of
HSPU: 7
Burpee Box Jump: 12

WEEK 41 - MON MAY 07 2012

PHASE II:
Games Track Athletes -
Active Rest + Power Hour

WARMUP:
4 Rounds of
:15 Jumping Jack
:15 Squat
:15 Mountain Climber
:15 Jump Squat
Then
Run/lunge 2x
Run/butt kickers 2x
Run/Straight Leg March 2x
Run/power skips 2x
Run/Spidey 2x
Run/Toes Hold 2x
Run/inchworm 2x
Then 4 Rounds of
:15 Plank
:15 Superman
:15 Side Plank - L
:15 Side Plank - R

EQUIPMENT:
DB #35/#25;
Dynamax #20/#14

WOD:
Two Partners
Burpee 1-10 x 1
Push Press 2-20 x 2
Pull Up 1-10 x 1
Wall Ball 2-20 x 2
For time

GAMES: REST DAY

POWER HOUR:
NOTE: All lifts EMOTM
BSQ 5-5-5-5-5

WEEK 41 - TUE MAY 08 2012

PHASE II:
Games Track Athletes - All

WARMUP:
4 Rounds of
:15 Jumping Jack
:15 Squat
:15 Mountain Climber
:15 Jump Squat
Then
Run/lunge 2x
Run/butt kickers 2x
Run/power skips 2x
Run/Spidey 2x
Run/inchworm 2x
Then 4 Rounds of
:15 Plank
:15 Superman
:15 Side Plank - L
:15 Side Plank - R

EQUIPMENT:
KB 24kg/16kg; Slammer #30/#20

WOD:
Row: 1000
Then American Swing & Ball Slam
21-15-9 for time

SKILL/DEV. WORK:
NOTE: IN ADDITION TO CLASS
Pull Up: 15
T2B : 15
3 Rounds (Completion)

GAMES WOD:
NOTE: IN ADDITION TO CLASS
DB SN: 1/1 x 5
Row: 150
3 Rounds for time

ACCESSORY:
NOTE: IN ADDITION TO CLASS
GHD Sit Up: 12
Swing: 12 (#124/88)
3 Rounds for time

POWER HOUR:
NOTE: IN ADDITION TO CLASS:
All lifts EMOTM
FSQ 5-5-5-5-5

WEEK 41 - WED MAY 09 2012

PHASE II:
Games Track Athletes - All

WARMUP:
4 Rounds of
:15 Jumping Jack
:15 Squat
:15 Mountain Climber
:15 Jump Squat
Then
Run/lunge 2x
Run/butt kickers 2x
Run/Straight Leg March 2x
Run/power skips 2x
Run/Spidey 2x
Run/Toes Hold 2x
Run/inchworm 2x
Then 4 Rounds of
:15 Plank
:15 Superman
:15 Side Plank - L
:15 Side Plank - R

EQUIPMENT: DB #35/#25

WOD:
Run: 100
Burpee: 7
Thruster: 7
AMRAP: 4 Minutes - Rest 1:00
- 4 Rounds

SKILL/DEV. WORK:
NOTE: IN ADDITION TO CLASS
Pistol: 1R/1L x 15

GAMES WOD:
NOTE: IN ADDITION TO CLASS
Shoulder to Overhead: 15
FSQ: 15
3 Rounds for time - BB #135/#95

POWER HOUR:
NOTE: IN ADDITION TO CLASS
All lifts EMOTM
PCL: 1 + 1 x 10

WEEK 41 -
THU MAY 10 2012

PHASE II:
Games Track Athletes -
Active Rest

WARMUP:
4 Rounds of
:15 Jumping Jack
:15 Squat
:15 Mountain Climber
:15 Jump Squat
Then
Run/lunge 2x
Run/butt kickers 2x
Run/Straight Leg March 2x
Run/power skips 2x
Run/Spidey 2x
Run/Toes Hold 2x
Run/inchworm 2x
Then 4 Rounds of
:15 Plank
:15 Superman
:15 Side Plank - L
:15 Side Plank - R

EQUIPMENT: Butcher #70/#50

WOD:
P1: Butcher Hi Push 25yds
P2: Butcher Lo Push 25yds
P3: Butcher Hi Push 25yds
Cycle Through
AMRAP: 12 Minutes

GAMES: ACTIVE REST DAY

SKILL/DEV. WORK:
Row/Roll prep

POWER HOUR:
NOTE: All lifts EMOTM
PSN: 1 + 1 x 10

WEEK 41 -
FRI MAY 11 2012

PHASE II:
Games Track Athletes - All

WARMUP:
4 Rounds of
:15 Jumping Jack
:15 Squat
:15 Mountain Climber
:15 Jump Squat
Then
Run/lunge 2x
Run/butt kickers 2x
Run/Straight Leg March 2x
Run/power skips 2x
Run/Spidey 2x
Run/Toes Hold 2x
Run/inchworm 2x
Then 4 Rounds of
:15 Plank
:15 Superman
:15 Side Plank - L
:15 Side Plank - R

EQUIPMENT:
DB #35/25

WOD:
Lunge (High Carry): 25yds
Push Press: 10
Push Up: 10
AMRAP: 7 Minutes - Rest 3:00
- 2 Rounds

**WEEK 41 -
SAT MAY 12 2012**

PHASE II:
Games Track Athletes - All

WARMUP:
4 Rounds of
:15 Jumping Jack
:15 Squat
:15 Mountain Climber
:15 Jump Squat
Then 4 Rounds of
:15 Plank
:15 Superman
:15 Side Plank - L
:15 Side Plank - R

EQUIPMENT:
BB #135/#95

WOD:
Amanda

Week 42

	SUNDAY 5/13	MONDAY 5/14	TUESDAY 5/15
WARM UP	**4 Rounds of** :15 Jumping Jack :15 Squat :15 MC :15 Jump Squat	**4 Rounds of** :15 Jumping Jack :15 Squat :15 MC :15 Jump Squat **Then** Run/lunge 2x Run/butt kickers 2x Run/Straight Leg March 2x Run/power skips 2x Run/Spidey 2x Run/Cartwheel 2x Run/Toes Hold 2x Run/inchworm 2x **Then 4 Rounds of** :15 Plank :15 Superman :15 Side Plank /L :15 Side Plank /R	**4 Rounds of** :15 Jumping Jack :15 Squat :15 MC :15 Jump Squat **Then** Run/lunge 2x Run/butt kickers 2x Run/Straight Leg March 2x Run/power skips 2x Run/Spidey 2x Run/Cartwheel 2x Run/Toes Hold 2x Run/inchworm 2x **Then 4 Rounds of** :15 Plank :15 Superman :15 Side Plank /L :15 Side Plank /R
EQUIPMENT	BB: 135/95		BB: 135/95 Dynamax #20/#14
WOD	DL: 5 CL: 5 FSQ: 5 PJ: 5 BSQ: 5 **AMRAP: 7 Minutes -** **Rest 3:00 - 3 Rounds**	**A1** : Burpee: 6 **A2** : HR Push Up (Score) **A3** : Air Squat (Score) **AMRAP: 12 Minutes**	Run: 200 Muscle Up: 3 Push Press: 6 Wall Ball: 9 **AMRAP: 5 Minutes -** **Rest 1:00 - 3 Rounds**
LIFTING/SKILL			
GAMES Phase II	Rest	Rest	Rest
SKILL/DEV WORK		Do something to recover. No pressure. STAY OUT OF THE GYM	Do something to recover. No pressure. STAY OUT OF THE GYM
GAMES WOD			
POWER HOUR			

WEDNESDAY 5/16	THURSDAY 5/17	FRIDAY 5/18	SATURDAY 5/19
4 Rounds of	**4 Rounds of**	**4 Rounds of**	**4 Rounds of**
:15 Jumping Jack	:15 Jumping Jack	:15 Jumping Jack	:15 Jumping Jack
:15 Squat	:15 Squat	:15 Squat	:15 Squat
:15 MC	:15 MC	:15 MC	:15 MC
:15 Jump Squat	:15 Jump Squat	:15 Jump Squat	:15 Jump Squat
Then	**Then**	**Then**	**Then 4 Rounds of**
Run/lunge 2x	Run/lunge 2x	Run/lunge 2x	:15 Plank
Run/butt kickers 2x	Run/butt kickers 2x	Run/butt kickers 2x	:15 Superman
Run/Straight Leg	Run/Straight Leg	Run/Straight Leg March 2x	:15 Side Plank /L
March 2x	March 2x	Run/power skips 2x	:15 Side Plank /R
Run/power skips 2x	Run/power skips 2x	Run/Spidey 2x	
Run/Spidey 2x	Run/Spidey 2x	Run/Cartwheel 2x	
Run/Cartwheel 2x	Run/Cartwheel 2x	Run/Toes Hold 2x	
Run/Toes Hold 2x	Run/Toes Hold 2x	Run/inchworm 2x	
Run/inchworm 2x	Run/inchworm 2x	**Then 4 Rounds of**	
Then 4 Rounds of	**Then 4 Rounds of**	:15 Plank	
:15 Plank	:15 Plank	:15 Superman	
:15 Superman	:15 Superman	:15 Side Plank /L	
:15 Side Plank /L	:15 Side Plank /L	:15 Side Plank /R	
:15 Side Plank /R	:15 Side Plank /R		
BB	BB	KB 2 (24/16)	BB 95/65
CL&J **EMOTM for 15 Minutes** - Increase loading	PSN **EMOTM for 15 Minutes** - Increase loading	Run: 200 KB Step Up (to 20in box): 1R/1L x 5 (2x24kg/16kg) Box Jump: 10 **AMRAP: 7 Minutes - Rest 3:00 - Two Rounds**	*Fran*
			KB Swing: 12 **EMOTM Rounds** (124/88)
Rest	**Rest**	**All**	**All**
Do something to recover. No pressure. STAY OUT OF THE GYM	**Do something to recover. No pressure. STAY OUT OF THE GYM**	KBSN 1/1 x 10 (Technique) Handwalk: 40ft Pull Up: 10 x 3 Sets (w/#20 Vest) Dips: 10 x 3 Sets (w/#20 Vest) Rope Climb: 5	Double Under: 50 x 2 Sets HSPU: 10 x 3 Sets MuscleUp:(1Strict +1Kipping) x 10 for 2 Sets PSN: 2 x 10 Sets - **Touch and Go** - Increase Loading
		BSQ: 7 PJ : 7 **EMOTM for 5 Rounds**	FSQ: 7 SJ: 7 **EMOTM for 5 Rounds**
		Jump Squat: 5 (65/45) **EMOTM for 10 Minutes**	CL&J - **Prison Rules** - 2 Reps every :15 x 16 - 145/105

WEEK 42 -
SUN MAY 13 2012

PHASE II:
Games Track Athletes - Rest

WARMUP:
4 Rounds of
:15 Jumping Jack
:15 Squat
:15 Mountain Climber
:15 Jump Squat

EQUIPMENT:
BB: 135/95

WOD:
DL: 5
CL: 5
FSQ: 5
PJ: 5
BSQ: 5
AMRAP: 7 Minutes -
Rest: 3:00 - 3 Rounds

GAMES:
REST DAY

WEEK 42 -
MON MAY 14 2012

PHASE II:
Games Track Athletes - Rest

WARMUP:
4 Rounds of
:15 Jumping Jack
:15 Squat
:15 Mountain Climber
:15 Jump Squat
Then
Run/lunge 2x
Run/butt kickers 2x
Run/Straight Leg March 2x
Run/power skips 2x
Run/Spidey 2x
Run/Cartwheel 2x
Run/Toes Hold 2x
Run/inchworm 2x
Then 4 Rounds of
:15 Plank
:15 Superman
:15 Side Plank - L
:15 Side Plank - R

WOD:
P1: Burpee: 6
P2: Push Up: HR (Score)
P3: Air Squat (Score)

GAMES:
Note: Do something to recover.
No pressure.
STAY OUT OF THE GYM

WEEK 42 -
TUE MAY 15 2012

PHASE II:
Games Track Athletes - Rest

WARMUP:
4 Rounds of
:15 Jumping Jack
:15 Squat
:15 Mountain Climber
:15 Jump Squat
Then
Run/lunge 2x
Run/butt kickers 2x
Run/Straight Leg March 2x
Run/power skips 2x
Run/Spidey 2x
Run/Cartwheel 2x
Run/Toes Hold 2x
Run/inchworm 2x
Then 4 Rounds of
:15 Plank
:15 Superman
:15 Side Plank - L
:15 Side Plank - R

EQUIPMENT:
BB: 135/95; Dynamax #20/#14

WOD:
Run: 200
Muscle Up: 3
Push Press: 6
Wall Ball: 9
AMRAP: 5 Minutes -
Rest 1:00 - 3 Rounds

GAMES:
Note: Do something to recover.
No pressure.
STAY OUT OF THE GYM

WEEK 42 -
WED MAY 16 2012

PHASE II:
Games Track Athletes - Rest

WARMUP:
4 Rounds of
:15 Jumping Jack
:15 Squat
:15 Mountain Climber
:15 Jump Squat
Then
Run/lunge 2x
Run/butt kickers 2x
Run/Straight Leg March 2x
Run/power skips 2x
Run/Spidey 2x
Run/Cartwheel 2x
Run/Toes Hold 2x
Run/inchworm 2x
Then 4 Rounds of
:15 Plank
:15 Superman
:15 Side Plank - L
:15 Side Plank - R

EQUIPMENT: BB

WOD:
CL & J EMOTM for 15 Minutes
- Increase loading

GAMES:
Note: Do something to recover.
No pressure.
STAY OUT OF THE GYM

WEEK 42 -
THU MAY 17 2012

PHASE II:
Games Track Athletes - Rest

WARMUP:
4 Rounds of
:15 Jumping Jack
:15 Squat
:15 Mountain Climber
:15 Jump Squat
Then
Run/lunge 2x
Run/butt kickers 2x
Run/Straight Leg March 2x
Run/power skips 2x
Run/Spidey 2x
Run/Cartwheel 2x
Run/Toes Hold 2x
Run/inchworm 2x
Then 4 Rounds of
:15 Plank
:15 Superman
:15 Side Plank - L
:15 Side Plank - R

EQUIPMENT: BB

WOD:
PSN EMOTM for 15 Minutes -
Increase Loading

GAMES:
Note: Do something to recover.
No pressure.
STAY OUT OF THE GYM

WEEK 42 -
FRI MAY 18 2012

PHASE II:
Games Track Athletes - All

WARMUP:
4 Rounds of
:15 Jumping Jack
:15 Squat
:15 Mountain Climber
:15 Jump Squat
Then
Run/lunge 2x
Run/butt kickers 2x
Run/power skips 2x
Run/Spidey 2x
Run/inchworm 2x
Then 4 Rounds of
:15 Plank
:15 Superman
:15 Side Plank - L
:15 Side Plank - R

EQUIPMENT: KB 2 (24/16)

WOD:
Run: 200
Weighted Step Up: 1/1 x 5 - to
20inch box w/2 24kg/16kg
Box Jump: 10
AMRAP: 7 Minutes - Rest 3:00
- 2 Rounds

SKILL/DEV. WORK:
KBSN: 1/1 x 10 (Technique)
Handwalk: 40ft
Pull Up: 10 x 3 Sets (w/#20 Vest)
Dips: 10 x 3 Sets (w/#20 Vest)
Rope Climb: 5

GAMES WOD:
BSQ: 7
PJ: 7
EMOTM for 5 Rounds

ACCESSORY:
Jump Squat: 5 EMOTM for
10 Minutes (65/45)

WEEK 42 -
SAT MAY 19 2012

PHASE II:
Games Track Athletes - All

WARMUP:
4 Rounds of
:15 Jumping Jack
:15 Squat
:15 Mountain Climber
:15 Jump Squat
Then 4 Rounds of
:15 Plank
:15 Superman
:15 Side Plank - L
:15 Side Plank - R

EQUIPMENT: BB 95/65

WOD:
Fran

LIFTING/SKILL DEV:
KB Swing: 12 EMOTM (124/88)

SKILL/DEV. WORK:
Double Under: 50 x 2 Sets
HSPU: 10 x 3 Sets
Muscle Up: (1 Strict + 1 Kipping)
x 10 for 2 Sets
PSN: 2x10 Sets -Touch and Go -
Increase Loading

GAMES WOD:
FSQ: 7
SJ: 7
EMOTM for 5 Rounds

ACCESSORY:
CL&J - Prison Rules -
2 Reps every :15 x 16 (145/105)

NOTE:
TRANSITION TO PHASE III
May 20, 2012, marks the transition
to the PHASE III training schedule.
This schedule is as follows:
- Monday: Active Rest
- Tuesday: Work
- Wednesday: Work
- Thursday: Rest
  (Rolling and stretching only)
- Friday: Work
- Saturday: Work
- Sunday: Work
The changes matched the
expected training schedule for the
Games. We were very lucky: the
number of regular training days
coincided with the Games
requirement for 2012. The rest of
the programming is for our gym,
and for athletes not training for
the 2012 Games season.

Week 43

	SUNDAY 5/20	MONDAY 5/21	TUESDAY 5/22
WARM UP	**4 Rounds of** :15 Jumping Jack :15 Squat :15 MC :15 Jump Squat **Then** 30/20/30 w/Squat bands	**4 Rounds of** :15 Jumping Jack :15 Squat :15 MC :15 Jump Squat **Then** 30/20/30 w/Squat bands **Then 4 Rounds of** :15 Plank :15 Superman :15 Side Plank /L :15 Side Plank /R	**4 Rounds of** :15 Jumping Jack :15 Squat :15 MC :15 Jump Squat **Then** 30/20/30 w/Squat bands **Then 4 Rounds of** :15 Plank :15 Superman :15 Side Plank /L :15 Side Plank /R
EQUIPMENT	BB 185/120 KB: 24kg/16kg		BB: 95/65 KB: 24/16
WOD	PCL: 3 Pull Up: 6 Swing: 9 **E2M for 15 Rounds**	**A1**: Run 50yds **A2**: Push Up (Score) **A3**: Ball Slam (Score) **AMRAP: 12 min**	Push Press: 21 Burpee: 15 American Swing: 9 **4 Rounds for time**
LIFTING/SKILL		Swing: 12 **EMOTM for 7 min** - #124/#88 - Load to tolerance	Run 25yds Lunge 25yds **AMRAP: 10 min**
GAMES Phase III	All	Active Rest	All
SKILL/DEV WORK	L-Sit - :20/:10 x 8 Hand Walk: 40ft Ring Dip: 10 (#20 Vest) Pull Up: 10 (#20 Vest) **Dips and PU anyhow**	CHOICE	KB SN (1+Windmill R/L) x 10 - Load to tolerance Rope Climb: 5
GAMES WOD	OHS: 7 BP: 7 **EMOTM for 5 min @80% of 1RM**		DL: 7 Thruster: 7 **EMOTM for 5 min @80% of 1RM**
ACCESSORY	GHD Sit Up: 20 FSQ: 7 - #225/#155 **5 Rounds for time**		***Death By HSPU:*** 1 Strict Rep **EMOTM until failure**
POWER HOUR		Sled Drag 800yds **for time** (#135/#90)	CL from blocks: 2-2-2-2-2-2-2-2-2-2-2 **EMOTM** (Loading variable)

278

WEDNESDAY 5/23	THURSDAY 5/24	FRIDAY 5/25	SATURDAY 5/26
4 Rounds of :15 Jumping Jack :15 Squat :15 MC :15 Jump Squat **Then** 30/20/30 w/Squat bands **Then 4 Rounds of** :15 Plank :15 Superman :15 Side Plank /L :15 Side Plank /R	**4 Rounds of** :15 Jumping Jack :15 Squat :15 MC :15 Jump Squat **Then** 30/20/30 w/ Squat bands **Then 4 Rounds of** :15 Plank :15 Superman :15 Side Plank /L :15 Side Plank /R	**4 Rounds of** :15 Jumping Jack :15 Squat :15 MC :15 Jump Squat **Then** 30/20/30 w/Squat bands **Then 4 Rounds of** :15 Plank :15 Superman :15 Side Plank /L :15 Side Plank /R	**4 Rounds of** :15 Jumping Jack :15 Squat :15 MC :15 Jump Squat **Then** 30/20/30 w/Squat bands **Then 4 Rounds of** :15 Plank :15 Superman :15 Side Plank /L :15 Side Plank /R
BB 185/120		KB 40kg/24kg BB #135/#95	BB 135/95
FSQ **(from ground)** Muscle Up **10, 9, 8, 7, 6, 5, 4, 3, 2, 1 for time**	*Cindy*	Swing: 21 T2B: 15 Thruster: 9 **3 Rounds for time**	*Elizabeth*
	Swing: 12 **EMOTM** **for 7 min -** #124/#88 - Load to tolerance		Sprint: 100 Jog: 100 **AMRAP: 10 min**
All + Olift	**Rest**	**All**	**All + Olift**
TGU: 1R/1L x 10 T2B: 10 x 5 Sets **Then** Ring Hold Top Ring Hold Bottom **:20/:10 x 16 Alternating**	Roll, recover, meditate etc.	BB Complex DL+CL+FSQ+PP+PJ+BSQ +OHS+SN -**2 Reps of each - 5 Rounds - Practice and refine movements**- Loading: 135/95 or as needed.	MU: (1 Strict+1 Kipping) x 10 Rounds
BSQ: Max Reps for 1:00 **Rest 1:00 - 10 Rounds** - #185/#135		FSQ: 5 SJ: 5 **EMOTM for 5 min** @80% of 1RM	OHS: 5 BP: 5 **EMOTM for 5 min** @80% of 1RM
Swing: 12 (#124/#88) Burpee: 12 **5 Rounds for time**		Butcher HiPush: 25yds Butcher LoPush: 25yds **E2M for 10 Rounds**(#90/#70)	Sled Drag 200yds (165/110) Run: 400yds **AMRAP: 20 min**
SN from Blocks: 2-2-2-2-2-2-2-2-2-2 **EMOTM** (Loading Variable)	Butcher HiPush: 25yds #180/120 Run 50yds **AMRAP: 20 min**		

WEEK 43 - SUN MAY 20 2012

PHASE III:

WARMUP:
4 Rounds of
:15 Jumping Jack
:15 Squat
 0 w/Squat bands

EQUIPMENT:
BB 185/120; KB: 24kg/16kg

WOD:
PCL: 3
Pull Up: 6
Swing: 9
E2M for 15 Rounds

SKILL/DEV. WORK:
NOTE: IN ADDITION TO CLASS
L-Sit - :20/:10 x 8
Hand Walk: 40ft
Ring Dip: 10 (#20 Vest)
Pull Up: 10 (#20 Vest)
Dips and Pull Ups
are anyhow

GAMES WOD:
NOTE: IN ADDITION TO CLASS
OHS: 7
BP: 7
EMOTM for 5 Rounds

ACCESSORY:
NOTE: IN ADDITION TO CLASS
GHD Sit Up: 20
FSQ: 7
5 Rounds for time -
#225/#155

WEEK 43 - MON MAY 21 2012

PHASE III:

WARMUP:
4 Rounds of
:15 Jumping Jack
:15 Squat
:15 Mountain Climber
:15 Jump Squat
Then
30/20/30 w/Squat bands
Then 4 Rounds of
:15 Plank
:15 Superman
:15 Side Plank - L
:15 Side Plank - R

WOD:
P1: Run 50yds
P2: Push Up (Score)
P3: Ball Slam (Score)
AMRAP: 12 Minutes

LIFTING/SKILL DEV:
Swing: 12 EMOTM for 7 Rounds
- #124/#88 (Load to tolerance)

SKILL/DEV. WORK:
CHOICE

GAMES:
ACTIVE REST DAY

POWER HOUR:
Sled Drag: 800yds (#135/#90) -
for time

WEEK 43 -
TUE MAY 22 2012

PHASE III:

WARMUP:
4 Rounds of
:15 Jumping Jack
:15 Squat
:15 Mountain Climber
:15 Jump Squat
Then
30/20/30 w/Squat bands
Then 4 Rounds of
:15 Plank
:15 Superman
:15 Side Plank - L
:15 Side Plank - R

EQUIPMENT:
BB: 95/65; KB: 24/16

WOD:
Push Press: 21
Burpee: 15
American Swing: 9
4 Rounds for time

LIFTING/SKILL DEV:
Run: 25yds
Lunge: 25yds
AMRAP: 10 Minutes

SKILL/DEV. WORK:
NOTE: IN ADDITION TO CLASS
KB SN: 1 + Windmill R/L x 10 -
Load to tolerance
Rope Climb: 5

GAMES WOD:
NOTE: IN ADDITION TO CLASS
DL: 7
Thruster: 7
EMOTM for 5 Rounds

ACCESSORY:
NOTE: IN ADDITION TO CLASS
Death By HSPU (Strict):
1 rep EMOTM for as long as capable

POWER HOUR:
NOTE: IN ADDITION TO CLASS
CL from blocks:
2-2-2-2-2-2-2-2-2-2-2 EMOTM
(Loading variable)

WEEK 43 -
WED MAY 23 2012

PHASE III:

WARMUP:
4 Rounds of
:15 Jumping Jack
:15 Squat
:15 Mountain Climber
:15 Jump Squat
Then
30/20/30 w/Squat bands
Then 4 Rounds of
:15 Plank
:15 Superman
:15 Side Plank - L
:15 Side Plank - R

EQUIPMENT: BB 185/120

WOD:
FSQ (from ground)
Muscle Up
10, 9, 8, 7, 6, 5, 4, 3, 2, 1 for time

SKILL/DEV. WORK:
*NOTE: IN ADDITION TO
CLASS AND O-LIFTING*
TGU: 1/1 x 10
T2B: 10 x 5 Sets
Then
Ring Hold Top
Ring Hold Bottom
:20/10 x 16 Alternating

GAMES WOD:
*NOTE: IN ADDITION TO
CLASS AND O-LIFTING*
BSQ: Max Reps for 1:00 -
Rest 1:00 - 10 Rounds -
#185/#135

ACCESSORY:
*NOTE: IN ADDITION TO
CLASS AND O-LIFTING*
Swing: 12 (#124/#88)
Burpee: 12
5 Rounds for time

POWER HOUR:
*NOTE: IN ADDITION TO
CLASS AND O-LIFTING*
SN from Blocks
2-2-2-2-2-2-2-2-2-2-2 EMOTM
(Loading Variable)

WEEK 43 -
THU MAY 24 2012

PHASE III:

WARMUP:
4 Rounds of
:15 Jumping Jack
:15 Squat
:15 Mountain Climber
:15 Jump Squat
Then
30/20/30 w/Squat bands
Then 4 Rounds of
:15 Plank
:15 Superman
:15 Side Plank - L
:15 Side Plank - R

WOD:
Cindy

LIFTING/SKILL DEV:
Swing: 12 EMOTM for
7 Rounds
(#124/#88)
Load to tolerance

SKILL/DEV. WORK:
Roll, recover, meditate etc.

GAMES:
REST DAY

POWER HOUR:
Butcher Hi Push: 25yds
- #180/120
Run: 50yds
AMRAP: 20 Minutes

WEEK 43 -
FRI MAY 25 2012

PHASE III:

WARMUP:
4 Rounds of
:15 Jumping Jack
:15 Squat
:15 Mountain Climber
:15 Jump Squat
Then
30/20/30 w/Squat bands
Then 4 Rounds of
:15 Plank
:15 Superman
:15 Side Plank - L
:15 Side Plank - R

EQUIPMENT:
KB 40kg/24kg; BB #135/#95

WOD:
Swing: 21
T2B: 15
Thruster: 9
3 Rounds for time

SKILL/DEV. WORK:
NOTE: IN ADDITION TO CLASS
BB Complex:
DL+CL+FSQ+PP+PJ+BSQ+
OHS+SN - 2 Reps of each
- 5 Rounds
Practice and refine movements
- Loading: 135/95 or as needed.

GAMES WOD:
NOTE: IN ADDITION TO CLASS
FSQ: 5
SJ: 5
EMOTM for 5 Rounds

ACCESSORY:
NOTE: IN ADDITION TO CLASS
Butcher Hi-Push: 25yds
Butcher Low Push: 25yds
E2M for 10 Rounds - (#90/#70)

WEEK 43 -
SAT MAY 26 2012

PHASE III:

WARMUP:
4 Rounds of
:15 Jumping Jack
:15 Squat
:15 Mountain Climber
:15 Jump Squat
Then
30/20/30 w/Squat bands
Then 4 Rounds of
:15 Plank
:15 Superman
:15 Side Plank - L
:15 Side Plank - R

EQUIPMENT: BB 135/95

WOD:
Elizabeth

LIFTING/SKILL DEV:
Sprint: 100
Jog: 100
AMRAP: 10 Minutes

SKILL/DEV. WORK:
*NOTE: IN ADDITION TO
CLASS AND O-LIFTING*
MU: 1 (Strict) + 1 (Kipping)
- 10 Rounds

GAMES WOD:
*NOTE: IN ADDITION TO
CLASS AND O-LIFTING*
OHS: 5
BP: 5
EMOTM for 5 Rounds

ACCESSORY:
*NOTE: IN ADDITION TO
CLASS AND O-LIFTING*
Sled Drag: 200yds - #165/#110
Run: 400yds
AMRAP: 20 Minutes

Week 44

	SUNDAY 5/27	MONDAY 5/28	TUESDAY 5/29
WARM UP	Run: 400 30/20/30 w/Bands	Run: 400 30/20/30 w/Bands	Run: 400 30/20/30 w/Bands
EQUIPMENT	Slammer 40/30 DL: 155/105		DB (2) #35/#25
WOD	Ball Slam: 10 DL: 12 Run: 200 **AMRAP: 20 min**	*Murph*	DBHCL: 3 DBFSQ: 3 DBSJ: 3 Run: 200 **AMRAP: 17 min**
LIFTING/SKILL		Really?	Swing: 12 **EMOTM for 7 min** - #124/#88 (Load to tolerance)
GAMES Phase III	All	Class Only	All
SKILL/DEV WORK			TGU: 1R/1L x 10 T2B: 10 x 5 Sets **Then** Ring Hold Top Ring Hold Bottom **:20/:10 x 16 Alternating**
GAMES WOD	BSQ: 5 PJ: 5 **EMOTM for 5 min** @80% of 1RM		DL: 5 TH: 5 **EMOTM for 5 min** @80% of 1RM
ACCESSORY			Butcher HiPush: 25yds (180/120) Run: 50yds **AMRAP: 15 min**
POWER HOUR			SNBAL: 2 x 10 Sets - Work up in loading

284

WEDNESDAY 5/30	THURSDAY 5/31	FRIDAY 6/1	SATURDAY 6/2
4 Rounds of :15 Jumping Jack :15 Squat :15 Jump Squat	Run: 400 30/20/30 w/Bands	**4 Rounds of** :15 Jumping Jack :15 Squat :15 MC :15 Jump Squat	**4 Rounds of** :15 Jumping Jack :15 Squat :15 MC :15 Jump Squat
BB 65/45		BB 135/95	BB 45/35
Thruster Jumping Pull Ups **21, 15, 9 for time - 3:00** **Cap - Rest 2:00 - 5** **Rounds**	**2-Partner WOD** Swing: 2-20 by 2 Thruster: 1-10 by 1 Push Press: 2-20 by 2 Pull Up: 1-10 by 1 **For time**	Run: 200 SN: 3 MU: 3 **AMRAP: 30 min**	*Jackie*
			Run: 100 Burpee: 10 **AMRAP: 10 min**
All+ O-Lifting	**Rest**	**All**	**All + O-Lifting**
L-Sit - :20/:10 x 8 Hand Walk: 40ft Ring Dip: 10 (#20 Vest) Pull Up: 10 (#20 Vest) **Dips and PU anyhow**		L-Sit - :20/:10 x 8 Hand Walk: 40ft Ring Dip: 10 (#20 Vest) Pull Up: 10 (#20 Vest) **Dips and PU anyhow**	KB SN (1+Windmill R/L) x 10 - Load to tolerance Rope Climb: 5
FSQ: Max Reps for 1:00 - **Rest 1:00 - 10 Rounds -** (175/115)		BSQ: 3 PJ: 3 **EMOTM for 5 min** @90% of 1RM	FSQ: 3 SJ: 3 **EMOTM for 5 min** @90% of 1RM
Swing: 3 Reps every :15 for 16 intervals - 124/88		Row: 500 - **Rest 1:00 - 5** **Rounds - Men: 1:45 -** **Women 1:55 - If you miss** **the time, repeat the** **interval - 10 interval limit.**	Sled Drag: 200yds - #165/110 Run: 400yds **AMRAP: 20 min**

**WEEK 44 -
SUN MAY 27 2012**

PHASE III:

WARMUP:
Run: 400
30/20/30 w/bands

EQUIPMENT:
Slammer 40/30; DL: 155/105

WOD:
Ball Slam: 10
DL: 12
Run: 200
AMRAP: 20 Minute

GAMES WOD:
NOTE: IN ADDITION TO CLASS
BSQ: 5
PJ: 5
EMOTM

**WEEK 44 -
MON MAY 28 2012**

PHASE III:

WARMUP:
Run: 400
30/20/30

WOD:
Murph

LIFTING/SKILL DEV:
Really?

WEEK 44 - TUE MAY 29 2012

PHASE III:

WARMUP:
Run: 400
30/20/30 w/Bands

EQUIPMENT:
DB (2) #35/#25

WOD:
DBHCL: 3
DBFSQ: 3
DBSJ: 3
Run: 200
AMRAP: 17 Minutes

LIFTING/SKILL DEV:
Swing: 12 EMOTM for
7 Rounds (#124/#88)
Load to tolerance

SKILL/DEV. WORK:
NOTE: IN ADDITION TO CLASS
TGU: 1/1 x 10
T2B: 10 x 5 Sets
Then
Ring Hold Top
Ring Hold Bottom
:20/10 x 16 Alternating

GAMES WOD:
NOTE: IN ADDITION TO CLASS
DL: 5
TH: 5
EMOTM

ACCESSORY:
NOTE: IN ADDITION TO CLASS
Butcher Hi Push: 25yds - (180/120)
Run: 50yds
AMRAP: 15 Minutes

POWER HOUR:
NOTE: IN ADDITION TO CLASS
SNBAL: 2 reps x 10 Sets -
Work up in loading

WEEK 44 - WED MAY 30 2012

PHASE III:

WARMUP:
4 Rounds of
:15 Jumping Jack
:15 Squat
:15 Mountain Climber
:15 Jump Squat

EQUIPMENT:
BB 65/45

WOD:
Thruster
Jumping Pull Ups
21, 15, 9 for time - 3:00 Cap -
Rest 2:00 - 5 Rounds

SKILL/DEV. WORK:
*NOTE: IN ADDITION TO
CLASS AND O-LIFTING*
L-Sit - :20/:10 x 8
Hand Walk: 40ft
Ring Dip: 10 (#20 Vest)
Pull Up: 10 (#20 Vest)
Dips and Pull Ups are anyhow

GAMES WOD:
*NOTE: IN ADDITION TO
CLASS AND O-LIFTING*
FSQ: Max Reps for 1:00 -
Rest 1:00 - 10 Rounds
(175/115)

ACCESSORY:
*NOTE: IN ADDITION TO
CLASS AND O-LIFTING*
Swing: 3 Reps every :15 for
16 intervals - #124/#88

WEEK 44 -
THU MAY 31 2012

PHASE III:

WARMUP:
Run: 400
30/20/30 w/Bands

WOD:
Partner WOD
Swing: 2-20 by 2
Thruster: 1-10 by 1
Push Press: 2-20 by 2
Pull Up: 1-10 by 1
For time

GAMES:
REST DAY

WEEK 44 -
FRI JUN 01 2012

PHASE III:

WARMUP:
4 Rounds of
:15 Jumping Jack
:15 Squat
:15 Mountain Climber
:15 Jump Squat

EQUIPMENT:
BB 135/95

WOD:
Run: 200
SN: 3
MU: 3
AMRAP: 30 Minutes

SKILL/DEV. WORK:
NOTE: IN ADDITION TO CLASS
L-Sit - :20/:10 x 8
Hand Walk: 40ft
Ring Dip: 10 (#20 Vest)
Pull Up: 10 (#20 Vest)
Dips and Pull Ups are anyhow

GAMES WOD:
NOTE: IN ADDITION TO CLASS
BSQ: 3
PJ: 3
EMOTM

ACCESSORY:
NOTE: IN ADDITION TO CLASS
Row: 500 - Rest 1:00 - 5 Rounds
Men: 1:45 - Women 1:55 -
If you miss the time,
repeat the interval - 10 interval limit

WEEK 44 -
SAT JUN 02 2012

PHASE III:

WARMUP:
4 Rounds of
:15 Jumping Jack
:15 Squat
:15 Mountain Climber
:15 Jump Squat

EQUIPMENT:
BB 45/35

WOD:
Jackie

LIFTING/SKILL DEV:
Run: 100
Burpee: 10
AMRAP: 10 Minutes

SKILL/DEV. WORK:
*NOTE: IN ADDITION TO
CLASS AND O-LIFTING*
KB SN: 1 + Windmill R/L x 10
(Load to tolerance)
Rope Climb: 5

GAMES WOD:
*NOTE: IN ADDITION TO
CLASS AND O-LIFTING*
FSQ: 3
SJ: 3
EMOTM

ACCESSORY:
*NOTE: IN ADDITION TO
CLASS AND O-LIFTING*
Sled Drag: 200yds - #165/110
Run: 400yds
AMRAP: 20 Minutes

Week 45

	SUNDAY 6/3	MONDAY 6/4	TUESDAY 6/5
WARM UP	**4 Rounds of** :15 Jumping Jack :15 Squat :15 MC :15 Jump Squat	Run/lunge 2x Run/butt kickers 2x Run/Straight Leg March 2x Run/power skips 2x Run/Spidey 2x Run/Toes Hold 2x Run/inchworm 2x 30/20/30 w/bands	**4 Rounds of** :15 Jumping Jack :15 Squat :15 MC :15 Jump Squat
EQUIPMENT	BB: 135/95 BB: 225/155	Dynamax #20/#14	BB: 115/75
WOD	Thruster: 7 Deadlift: 12 **3 Rounds for time**	*Karen*	*Tabata* - :20/:10 x 8 - **Rest 1:00** Air Squat Push Press AbMat Sit Up SDLHP PCL **Score total reps for each exercise**
GAMES Phase III	All	Skill/Dev Only	All
SKILL/DEV WORK	L-Sit - :20/:10 x 8 Hand Walk: 40ft Ring Dip: 10 (#20 Vest) Pull Up: 10 (#20 Vest) **Dips and PU anyhow**	Swim/Bike/Etc.	TGU: 1R/1L x 10 T2B: 10 x 5 Sets **Then** Ring Hold Top Ring Hold Bottom **:20/:10 x 16 Alternating**
GAMES WOD	DL: 3 TH: 3 **EMOTM for 5 min** @90% of 1RM		OHS: 3 BP: 3 **EMOTM for 5 min** @90% of 1RM
ACCESSORY	CL+FSQ+J **EMOTM for 20 min** (#200/130)		Butcher HiPush: 50yds (180/120) Slam: 15 #40/#30 Run: 50yds **AMRAP: 20 min**
POWER HOUR			PSN+SNBAL+SN **EMOTM for 15 min**

WEDNESDAY 6/6	THURSDAY 6/7	FRIDAY 6/8	SATURDAY 6/9
Run/lunge 2x Run/butt kickers 2x Run/Straight Leg March 2x Run/power skips 2x Run/Spidey 2x Run/Toes Hold 2x Run/inchworm 2x 30/20/30 w/bands	**4 Rounds of** :15 Jumping Jack :15 Squat :15 MC :15 Jump Squat	Run/lunge 2x Run/butt kickers 2x Run/Straight Leg March 2x Run/power skips 2x Run/Spidey 2x Run/Toes Hold 2x Run/inchworm 2x 30/20/30 w/bands	**4 Rounds of** :15 Jumping Jack :15 Squat :15 MC :15 Jump Squat
Box: 24/20	Butcher 70/50	BB: 115/75	
Box Jump: 12 Pull Up: 10 **5 Rounds for time**	**A1** : Butcher HiPush **A2** : Butcher LoPush **A3** : Butcher HiPush **Rotate through for duration - AMRAP: 12 min**	PSN: 8 T2B: 8 Ring Push Up: 8 **AMRAP: 8 min - Rest 2:00 - 2 Rounds**	*CrossFit For Hope*
All + O lift	**Active Rest Day**	**All**	**All + O lift**
Run: 800 x 4 - **Rest 1:00** HSPU (Strict): 3 x 10 Sets (Regional Standard)		L-Sit - :20/:10 x 8 Hand Walk: 40ft Ring Dip: 10 (#20 Vest) Pull Up: 10 (#20 Vest) **Dips and PU anyhow**	KB SN (1+Windmill R/L) x 10 - Load to tolerance Rope Climb: 5
DL: 7 (345/225) MU: 7 Wall Ball: 21 (#20/14) **3 Rounds for time**		BSQ: 7 PJ: 7 **EMOTM for 5 min @80%** of 1RM	FSQ: 7 SJ: 7 **EMOTM for 5 min @80%** of 1RM
Swing: 3 reps every :15 for 16 intervals - 124/88		CL&J - **Prison Rules** - 2 reps every :15 x 16 Intervals - 155/105	PSN - **Prison Rules** - 2 reps every :15 x 16 Intervals - 155/105
	Pull Up (Strict): 3 Reg/Nar/Wide/Rev/MC-L/MC-R Dips (Strict): 3 **Alternate - completion**		

WEEK 45 -
SUN JUN 03 2012

PHASE III:

WARMUP:
4 Rounds of
:15 Jumping Jack
:15 Squat
:15 Mountain Climber
:15 Jump Squat

EQUIPMENT:
BB: 135/95; BB: 225/155

WOD:
Thruster: 7
Deadlift: 12
3 Rounds for time

LIFTING/SKILL DEV:
Swing: 12 Reps EMOTM
for 7 Sets - #124/#88 or heavy load

SKILL/DEV. WORK:
NOTE: IN ADDITION TO CLASS
L-Sit - :20/:10 x 8
Hand Walk: 40ft
Ring Dip: 10 (#20 Vest)
Pull Up: 10 (#20 Vest)
Dips and Pull Ups are anyhow

GAMES WOD:
NOTE: IN ADDITION TO CLASS
DL: 3
TH: 3
EMOTM

ACCESSORY:
NOTE: IN ADDITION TO CLASS
CL + FSQ + J EMOTM for
20 Minutes (#200/130)

WEEK 45 -
MON JUN 04 2012

PHASE III:

WARMUP:
Run/lunge 2x
Run/butt kickers 2x
Run/Straight Leg March 2x
Run/power skips 2x
Run/Spidey 2x
Run/Toes Hold 2x
Run/inchworm 2x
30/20/30 w/bands

EQUIPMENT:
Dynamax #20/#14

WOD:
Karen

GAMES:
ACTIVE REST DAY

SKILL/DEV. WORK:
Swim/Bike/Etc.

292

WEEK 45 - TUE JUN 05 2012

PHASE III:

WARMUP:
4 Rounds of
:15 Jumping Jack
:15 Squat
:15 Mountain Climber
:15 Jump Squat

EQUIPMENT: BB: 115/75

WOD:
Tabata :20/:10 x 8 - Rest 1:00
Air Squat
Push Press
AbMat Sit Up
SDLHP
PCL
Score total reps for each exercise

LIFTING/SKILL DEV:
Muscle Transitions: 30 (from knees)

SKILL/DEV. WORK:
NOTE: IN ADDITION TO CLASS
TGU: 1/1 x 10
T2B: 10 x 5 Sets
Then
Ring Hold Top
Ring Hold Bottom
:20/10 x 16 Alternating

GAMES WOD:
NOTE: IN ADDITION TO CLASS
OHS: 3
BP: 3
EMOTM

ACCESSORY:
NOTE: IN ADDITION TO CLASS
Butcher Hi Push: 50yds (180/120)
Slam: 15 - #40/#30
Run: 50yds
AMRAP: 20 Minutes

POWER HOUR:
NOTE: IN ADDITION TO CLASS
PSN + SNBAL + SN
EMOTM for 15 Minutes

WEEK 45 - WED JUN 06 2012

PHASE III:

WARMUP:
Run/lunge 2x
Run/butt kickers 2x
Run/Straight Leg March 2x
Run/power skips 2x
Run/Spidey 2x
Run/Toes Hold 2x
Run/inchworm 2x
30/20/30 w/bands

EQUIPMENT:
Box: 24/20

WOD:
Box Jump: 12
Pull Up: 10
5 Rounds for time

SKILL/DEV. WORK:
NOTE: IN ADDITION TO CLASS AND O-LIFTING
Run: 800 - Rest 1:00 - 4 Intervals
HSPU (Strict): 3 Reps -
10 Sets (Regional Standard)

GAMES WOD:
NOTE: IN ADDITION TO CLASS AND O-LIFTING
DL: 7 (345/225)
MU: 7
Wall Ball: 21 (#20/14)
3 Rounds for time

ACCESSORY:
NOTE: IN ADDITION TO CLASS AND O-LIFTING
Swing: 3 Reps every :15
for 16 intervals - (124/88)

WEEK 45 -
THU JUN 07 2012

PHASE III:

WARMUP:
4 Rounds of
:15 Jumping Jack
:15 Squat
:15 Mountain Climber
:15 Jump Squat

EQUIPMENT:
Butcher 70/50

WOD:
P1: High Push
P2: Low Push
P3: High Push
Rotate through for duration
AMRAP: 12 Minutes

GAMES:
ACTIVE REST DAY

LIFTING/SKILL DEV:
Push Up: 10
Air Squat: 10
AMRAP: 7 Minutes

POWER HOUR:
Pull Up (Strict): 3 Reg/Nar/
Wide/Rev/MC-L/MC-R
Dips (Strict): 3
Alternate

WEEK 45 -
FRI JUN 08 2012

PHASE III:

WARMUP:
Run/lunge 2x
Run/butt kickers 2x
Run/Straight Leg March 2x
Run/power skips 2x
Run/Spidey 2x
Run/Toes Hold 2x
Run/inchworm 2x
Then
30/20/30 w/bands

EQUIPMENT:
BB: 115/75

WOD:
PSN: 8
T2B: 8
Ring Push Up: 8
AMRAP: 8 Minutes -
Rest 2:00 - 2 Rounds

LIFTING/SKILL DEV:
Run: 50yds every :30 for
20 Intervals

SKILL/DEV. WORK:
NOTE: IN ADDITION TO CLASS
L-Sit - :20/:10 x 8
Hand Walk: 40ft
Ring Dip: 10 (#20 Vest)
Pull Up: 10 (#20 Vest)
Dips and Pull Ups are anyhow

GAMES WOD:
NOTE: IN ADDITION TO CLASS
BSQ: 7
PJ: 7
EMOTM

ACCESSORY:
NOTE: IN ADDITION TO CLASS
CL&J - Prison Rules - 2 Reps
every :15 x 16 Intervals - 155/105

WEEK 45 -
SAT JUN 09 2012

PHASE III:

WARMUP:
4 Rounds of
:15 Jumping Jack
:15 Squat
:15 Mountain Climber
:15 Jump Squat

WOD:
CrossFit For Hope

SKILL/DEV. WORK:
NOTE: IN ADDITION TO
CLASS AND O-LIFTING
KB SN: 1 + Windmill R/L x 10
(Load to tolerance)
Rope Climb: 5

GAMES WOD:
NOTE: IN ADDITION TO
CLASS AND O-LIFTING
FSQ: 7
SJ: 7
EMOTM

ACCESSORY:
NOTE: IN ADDITION TO
CLASS AND O-LIFTING
PSN - Prison Rules - 2 Reps
every :15 x 16 Intervals - 155/105

Week 46

	SUNDAY 6/10	MONDAY 6/11	TUESDAY 6/12
WARM UP	Run/lunge 2x Run/butt kickers 2x Run/Straight Leg March 2x Run/power skips 2x Run/Spidey 2x Run/Toes Hold 2x Run/inchworm 2x 30/20/30 w/bands	Run/lunge 2x Run/butt kickers 2x Run/Straight Leg March 2x Run/power skips 2x Run/Spidey 2x Run/Toes Hold 2x Run/inchworm 2x 30/20/30 w/bands	Run: 400 30/20/30 w/Bands **Then 3 Rounds of** HCL: 3 Tall CL: 3 FSQ: 3 SJ: 3
EQUIPMENT	BB: 115/75	Slammer: #40/#30 Dynamax #20/#14	Loading Variable
W O D	Run: 800 Pull Up: 50 Push Press: 50 OHS: 50 Run: 800	Ball Slam: 12 Wall Ball: 12 Run: 200 **AMRAP: 20 Min**	CL+2FSQ+J **EMOTM for 20 Min**
LIFTING/SKILL	Swing: 12 **EMOTM for 7 Min** (#124/#88 or heavy bell)		Swing: 12 **EMOTM for 7 Min** (#124/#88 or heavy bell)
GAMES Phase III	All	Active Rest	All
SKILL/DEV WORK	L-Sit - :20/:10 x 8 Wall Walk to HSPU (Strict): 10	CHOICE	Rope Climb: 3 Run: 400 **3 Rounds for time**
GAMES W O D	DL: 7 TH: 7 **EMOTM for 10 Min** @80% of 1RM		OHS: 7 BP: 7 **EMOTM for 10 Min** @80% of 1RM
ACCESSORY	CL from Blocks: 2 **EMOTM for 10 Min** @60% of 1 RM Jerk from Blocks: 2 **EMOTM for 10 Min** @60% of 1 RM		SN from Blocks: 2 **EMOTM for 10 Min** @60% of 1 RM SNBAL from Blocks: 2 **EMOTM for 10 Min** @60% of 1 RM
POWER HOUR			HSN+OHS+SN: 10 Sets - Increase loading - **Work Skills**

WEDNESDAY 6/13	THURSDAY 6/14	FRIDAY 6/15	SATURDAY 6/16
4 Rounds of :15 Jumping Jack :15 Squat :15 MC :15 Jump Squat	Run/lunge 2x Run/butt kickers 2x Run/Straight Leg March 2x Run/power skips 2x Run/Spidey 2x Run/Toes Hold 2x Run/inchworm 2x 30/20/30 w/bands	**4 Rounds of** :15 Jumping Jack :15 Squat :15 MC :15 Jump Squat	**4 Rounds of** :15 Jumping Jack :15 Squat :15 MC :15 Jump Squat
BB: 115/75	KB: 24/16kg DB: 35/25	BB #115/#75	Dynamax #20/#14 Box 24/20
Thruster: 12 T2B: 12 **AMRAP: 3 Min -** **Rest 1:00 - 7** **Rounds**	Swing: 20 Push Press: 15 Burpee: 10 **AMRAP: 7 Min - Rest** **3:00 - 3 Rounds**	DL: 5 CL: 5 FSQ: 5 PJ: 5 **AMRAP: 45 Min (Yes,**	*Kelly*
		Swing: 12 **EMOTM for** **7 Min** (#124/#88 or heavy bell)	
All + O-Lift	**Rest Day**	**All**	**All + O-Lift**
TGU: 1R/1L x 10 T2B: 10 x 5 Sets **Then** Ring Hold Top Ring Hold Bottom **:20/:10 x 16** **Alternating**		MU: 3 **EMOTM for 10** **Min** w/#20 Vest	C2B PU: 12 w/#20 Burpee: 10 w/#20 **5 Rounds for time**
GHD Sit Up: 15 FSQ: 10 (185/135) **5 Rounds for time**		BSQ: 5 PJ: 5 **EMOTM for 10 Min** @80% of 1RM	FSQ: 5 SJ: 5 **EMOTM for 10 Min** @80% of 1RM
CL&J - **Prison Rules** - 2 reps every :15 x 16 Intervals - 155/105		Sled Pull: 200yds 155/100 Run: 200yds **AMRAP: 10 Min**	Butcher HiPush: 25yds 270/175 Run: 50 **AMRAP: 10 Min**

WEEK 46 - SUN JUN 10 2012

PHASE III:

WARMUP:
Run/lunge 2x
Run/butt kickers 2x
Run/Straight Leg March 2x
Run/power skips 2x
Run/Spidey 2x
Run/Toes Hold 2x
Run/inchworm 2x
30/20/30 w/bands

EQUIPMENT:
BB: 115/75

WOD:
Run: 800
Pull Up: 50
Push Press: 50
OHS: 50
Run: 800

LIFTING/SKILL DEV:
Swing: 12 EMOTM for 7 Sets
- #124/#88 or heavy bell

SKILL/DEV. WORK:
NOTE: IN ADDITION TO CLASS
L-Sit - :20/:10 x 8
Wall Walk to HSPU x 10 (Strict)

GAMES WOD:
NOTE: IN ADDITION TO CLASS
DL: 7
TH: 7
EMOTM for 10 Minutes

ACCESSORY:
NOTE: IN ADDITION TO CLASS
CL from Blocks: 2 EMOTM
for 10 Sets @60% of 1RM
Jerk from Blocks: 2 EMOTM
for 10 Sets @60% of 1RM

WEEK 46 - MON JUN 11 2012

PHASE III:

WARMUP:
Run/lunge 2x
Run/butt kickers 2x
Run/Straight Leg March 2x
Run/power skips 2x
Run/Spidey 2x
Run/Toes Hold 2x
Run/inchworm 2x
30/20/30 w/bands

EQUIPMENT:
Slammer: #40/#30;
Dynamax #20/#14

WOD:
Ball Slam: 12
Wall Ball: 12
Run: 200
AMRAP: 20 Minutes

GAMES:
ACTIVE REST DAY

SKILL/DEV. WORK:
CHOICE

WEEK 46 - TUE JUN 12 2012

PHASE III:

WARMUP:
Run: 400
30/20/30 w/Bands
Then 3 Rounds of
HCL: 3
Tall CL: 3
FSQ: 3
SJ: 3

EQUIPMENT: Loading Variable

WOD:
CL + 2xFSQ + J EMOTM
for 20 Minutes

LIFTING/SKILL DEV:
Swing: 12 EMOTM for 7 Sets
- #124/#88 or heavy bell

SKILL/DEV. WORK:
NOTE: IN ADDITION TO CLASS
Rope Climb: 3
Run: 400
3 Rounds for time

GAMES WOD:
NOTE: IN ADDITION TO CLASS
OHS: 7
BP: 7
EMOTM for 10 Minutes

ACCESSORY:
NOTE: IN ADDITION TO CLASS
SN from Block: 2 EMOTM for
10 Sets @60% of 1RM
SNBAL from Block: 2 EMOTM
for 10 Sets @60% of 1RM

POWER HOUR:
NOTE: IN ADDITION TO CLASS
HSN + OHS + SN for 10 Sets
- Increase loading - Work Skills

WEEK 46 - WED JUN 13 2012

PHASE III:

WARMUP:
4 Rounds of
:15 Jumping Jack
:15 Squat
:15 Mountain Climber
:15 Jump Squat

EQUIPMENT:
BB: 115/75

WOD:
Thruster: 12
T2B: 12
AMRAP: 3 Minutes -
Rest 1:00 - 7 Rounds

SKILL/DEV. WORK:
*NOTE: IN ADDITION TO CLASS
AND O-LIFTING*
TGU: 1/1 x 10
T2B: 10 x 5 Sets
Then
Ring Hold Top
Ring Hold Bottom
:20/10 x 16 Alternating

GAMES WOD:
*NOTE: IN ADDITION TO
CLASS AND O-LIFTING*
GHD Sit Up: 15
FSQ: 10 (185/135)
5 Rounds for time

ACCESSORY:
*NOTE: IN ADDITION TO CLASS
AND O-LIFTING*
CL&J - Prison Rules -
2 Reps every
:15 x 16 Intervals (155/105)

WEEK 46 - THU JUN 14 2012

PHASE III:

WARMUP:
Run/lunge 2x
Run/butt kickers 2x
Run/Straight Leg March 2x
Run/power skips 2x
Run/Spidey 2x
Run/Toes Hold 2x
Run/inchworm 2x
30/20/30 w/bands

EQUIPMENT:
KB: 24/16kg; DB: 35/25

WOD:
Swing: 20
Push Press: 15
Burpee: 10
AMRAP: 7 Minutes -
Rest 3:00 - 3 Rounds

GAMES:
REST DAY

WEEK 46 - FRI JUN 15 2012

PHASE III:

WARMUP:
4 Rounds of
:15 Jumping Jack
:15 Squat
:15 Mountain Climber
:15 Jump Squat

EQUIPMENT:
BB #115/#75

WOD:
DL: 5
CL: 5
FSQ: 5
PJ: 5
AMRAP: 45 Minutes
(Yes, 45 minutes)

LIFTING/SKILL DEV:
Swing: 12 EMOTM for 7 Sets -
#124/#88 or heavy bell

SKILL/DEV. WORK:
NOTE: IN ADDITION TO CLASS
Muscle Up: 3 EMOTM for
10 Sets (w/#20 Vest)

GAMES WOD:
NOTE: IN ADDITION TO CLASS
BSQ: 5
PJ: 5
EMOTM for 10 Minutes

ACCESSORY:
NOTE: IN ADDITION TO CLASS
Sled Pull: 200yds - (155/100)
Run: 200yds
AMRAP: 10 Minutes

WEEK 46 -
SAT JUN 16 2012

PHASE III:

WARMUP:
4 Rounds of
:15 Jumping Jack
:15 Squat
:15 Mountain Climber
:15 Jump Squat

EQUIPMENT:
Dynamax #20/#14; Box 24/20

WOD:
Kelly

SKILL/DEV. WORK:
NOTE: IN ADDITION TO
CLASS AND O-LIFTING
C2B PU: 12 (w/#20 Vest)
Burpee: 10 (w/#20 Vest)
5 Rounds for time

GAMES WOD:
NOTE: IN ADDITION TO
CLASS AND O-LIFTING
FSQ: 5
SJ: 5
EMOTM for 10 Minutes

ACCESSORY:
NOTE: IN ADDITION TO
CLASS AND O-LIFTING
Butcher: 25yds - (270/175)
Run: 50
AMRAP: 10 Minutes

NOTES

Week 47

	SUNDAY 6/17	MONDAY 6/18	TUESDAY 6/19
WARM UP	**4 Rounds of** :15 Jumping Jack :15 Squat :15 MC :15 Jump Squat **Then** 30/20/30 w/bands	Run: 400 **Then HSN** **Progression w/BB** **2 Rounds of** Dip/Catch: 3 Dip/Catch/OHS: 3 Dip/Hinge/Catch/ OHS: 3 Dip/Hinge/SN: 3	Run: 800 30/20/30 w/bands
EQUIPMENT	BB: 185/135	Loading variable based on ability	
WOD	Run: 400 BSQ: 12 **(from** **ground)** **3 Rounds for time**	HCL every :45 for 20 intervals	Burpee: 7 Run: 100 **EMOTM for 20 Min**
LIFTING/SKILL	Partner Sandbag Run: 50yds (#70/#50) **AMRAP: 12 Min -** **Alternating Partners**	*Tabata:* Air Squat Push Up AbMat **Cycle through** **continuous for 24** **intervals**	**5 Rounds (Strict) of** Dip: 10 DHPU: 10
GAMES **Phase III**	All	Active Rest	All
SKILL/DEV **WORK**	L-Sit - :20/:10 x 8 Wall Walk to HSPU (Strict): 10	CHOICE	Rope Climb: 3 Run: 400 **3 Rounds for time**
GAMES **WOD**	DL: 5 TH: 5 **EMOTM for 10 Min** **@80% of 1RM**		OHS: 5 BP: 5 **EMOTM for 10 Min** **@80% of 1RM**
ACCESSORY	KBSN: 1R/1L x 5 (28kg/20kg) Ball Slam: 12 #50/#40 **4 Rounds for time**		GHD Sit Up: 12 GHD Hip & Back Ext: 12 **5 Rounds** **(completion)**

WEDNESDAY 6/20	THURSDAY 6/21	FRIDAY 6/22	SATURDAY 6/23
4 Rounds of :15 Jumping Jack :15 Squat :15 MC :15 Jump Squat **Then 4 Rounds of** :15 Plank :15 Superman :15 Side Plank /L :15 Side Plank /R	Run: 400 **Then HSN** **Progression w/BB** **2 Rounds of** Dip/Catch: 3 Dip/Catch/FSQ: 3 Dip/Hinge/Catch/ FSQ: 3 Dip/Hinge/CL: 3	**4 Rounds of** :15 Jumping Jack :15 Squat :15 MC :15 Jump Squat **Then Review Skills w/BB** **3 Rounds of** PSN: 3 OSH: 3 SNBAL: 3	Run/lunge 2x Run/butt kickers 2x Run/Straight Leg March 2x Run/power skips 2x Run/Spidey 2x Run/Toes Hold 2x Run/inchworm 2x 30/20/30 w/bands
KB 28kg/20kg	Loading variable based on ability	BB #135/#95	
American Swing: 30 Pull up: 15 **3 Rounds for time**	HCL every :45 for 20 intervals	PSN: 7 OHS: 7 SNBAL: 7 **7 Rounds for time**	*Helen* (15 Min Cap)
Sprint: 50yds every :30 for 5 Min Sprint: 100yds every :30 for 5 min Sprint: 50yds every :30 for 5 min	Run Suicide (4 lengths) Burpees: 10yds **AMRAP: 12 Min**	MU Transition: 30 **for** **completion**	Swing: 12 **EMOTM** **for 7 Min** (#124/ #88)
All+O-Lift	**Rest Day**	**All**	**All +O-Lift**
TGU: 1R/1L x 10 T2B: 10 x 5 Sets **Then** Ring Hold Top Ring Hold Bottom **:20/:10 x 16 Alternating**		MU: 3 **EMOTM for 10 Min** w/#20 Vest L-Sit - :20/:10 x 8	C2B PU: 12 w/#20 Burpee: 10 w/#20 **5 Rounds for time**
Butcher Low Push: 50yds (70/50) Run: 50 **AMRAP: 12 Min**		BSQ: 3 PJ: 3 **EMOTM for 10 Min** @90% of 1RM	FSQ: 3 SJ: 3 **EMOTM for 10** **Min** @90% of 1RM
CL&J - **Prison Rules** - 2 reps every :15 x 16 Intervals - 155/105		Ring Dip T2B **10, 9, 8, 7, 6, 5, 4, 3, 2, 1** **for time**	

WEEK 47 -
SUN JUN 17 2012

PHASE III:

WARMUP:
4 Rounds of
:15 Jumping Jack
:15 Squat
:15 Mountain Climber
:15 Jump Squat
Then
30/20/30 w/bands

EQUIPMENT:
BB: 185/135

WOD:
Run: 400
BSQ: 12 (from ground)
3 Rounds for time

LIFTING/SKILL DEV:
Partner Sandbag Run:
50yds - (#70/#50)
AMRAP: 12 Minutes -
Alternating partners

SKILL/DEV. WORK:
NOTE: IN ADDITION TO CLASS
L-Sit - :20/:10 x 8
Wall Walk to HSPU x 10 (Strict)

GAMES WOD:
NOTE: IN ADDITION TO CLASS
DL: 5
TH: 5
EMOTM for 10 Minutes

ACCESSORY:
NOTE: IN ADDITION TO CLASS
KBSN: 1/1 x 5 (28kg/20kg)
Ball Slam: 12 - #50/#40
4 Round for time

WEEK 47 -
MON JUN 18 2012

PHASE III:

WARMUP:
Run: 400
Then
HSN Progression w/BB
2 Rounds of
Dip/Catch: 3
Dip/Catch/OHS: 3
Dip/Hinge/Catch/OHS: 3
Dip/Hinge/SN: 3

EQUIPMENT:
Loading variable based on
ability

WOD:
HSN: 1 every :45 for
20 intervals

LIFTING/SKILL DEV:
Tabata:
Air Squat
Push Up
AbMat
Cycle through continuous for
24 intervals

GAMES:
ACTIVE REST DAY

SKILL/DEV. WORK:
CHOICE

WEEK 47 - TUE JUN 19 2012

PHASE III:

WARMUP:
Run: 800
30/20/30 w/bands

WOD:
Burpee: 7
Run: 100
EMOTM for 20 Minutes

LIFTING/SKILL DEV:
5 Rounds (All Strict) of
Dip: 10
DHPU: 10

SKILL/DEV. WORK:
NOTE: IN ADDITION TO CLASS
Rope Climb: 3
Run: 400
3 Rounds for time

GAMES WOD:
NOTE: IN ADDITION TO CLASS
OHS: 5
BP: 5
EMOTM for 10 Minutes

ACCESSORY:
NOTE: IN ADDITION TO CLASS
GHD Sit Up: 12
GHD Hip & Back Ext: 12
5 Rounds for completion

WEEK 47 - WED JUN 20 2012

PHASE III:

WARMUP:
4 Rounds of
:15 Jumping Jack
:15 Squat
:15 Mountain Climber
:15 Jump Squat
Then 4 Rounds of
:15 Plank
:15 Superman
:15 Side Plank - L
:15 Side Plank - R

EQUIPMENT:
KB 28kg/20kg

WOD:
American Swing: 30
Pull up: 15
3 Rounds for time

LIFTING/SKILL DEV:
Sprint: 50yds every :30 for 5 Mins.
Sprint: 100yds every :30 for 5 Mins.
Sprint: 50yds every :30 for 5 Mins.

SKILL/DEV. WORK:
NOTE: IN ADDITION TO CLASS AND O-LIFTING
TGU: 1/1 x 10
T2B: 10 x 5 Sets
Then
Ring Hold Top
Ring Hold Bottom
:20/10 x 16 Alternating

GAMES WOD:
NOTE: IN ADDITION TO CLASS AND O-LIFTING
Butch Low Push: 50yds (70/50)
Run: 50
AMRAP: 12 Minutes

ACCESSORY:
NOTE: IN ADDITION TO CLASS AND O-LIFTING
CL&J - Prison Rules - 2 Reps every:
15 for 16 Intervals - 155/105

305

WEEK 47 - THU JUN 21 2012

PHASE III:

WARMUP:
Run: 400
Then
HCL Progression w/BB
2 Rounds of
Dip/Catch: 3
Dip/Catch/FSQ: 3
Dip/Hinge/Catch/FSQ: 3
Dip/Hinge/CL: 3

EQUIPMENT:
Loading variable based
on ability

WOD:
HCL: 1 every :45 for
20 intervals

LIFTING/SKILL DEV:
Run Suicide (4 Lengths)
10 Burpees
AMRAP: 12 Minutes

GAMES: REST DAY

WEEK 47 - FRI JUN 22 2012

PHASE III:

WARMUP:
4 Rounds of
:15 Jumping Jack
:15 Squat
:15 Mountain Climber
:15 Jump Squat
Then
w/BB 3 Rounds of
PSN: 3
OSH: 3
SNBAL: 3
Review skills

EQUIPMENT:
BB #135/#95

WOD:
PSN: 7
OHS: 7
SNBAL: 7
7 Rounds for time

LIFTING/SKILL DEV:
MU Transitions:
30 for completion

CONTINUED>>>>>>>>>

306

WEEK 47 -
FRI JUN 22 2012
CONTINUED

SKILL/DEV. WORK:
NOTE: IN ADDITION TO CLASS
Muscle Up: 3 EMOTM for 10 Sets (w/#20 Vest)
L-Sit - :20/:10 x 8

GAMES WOD:
NOTE: IN ADDITION TO CLASS
BSQ: 3
PJ: 3
EMOTM for 10 Minutes

ACCESSORY:
NOTE: IN ADDITION TO CLASS
Ring Dip
T2B
10, 9, 8, 7, 6, 5, 4, 3, 2, 1 for time

WEEK 47 -
SAT JUN 23 2012

PHASE III:

WARMUP:
Run/lunge 2x
Run/butt kickers 2x
Run/Straight Leg March 2x
Run/power skips 2x
Run/Spidey 2x
Run/Toes Hold 2x
Run/inchworm 2x
30/20/30 w/bands

WOD:
Helen (15 Minute Cap)

LIFTING/SKILL DEV:
Swing: 12 EMOTM for 7 Minutes (#124/#88)

SKILL/DEV. WORK:
NOTE: IN ADDITION TO CLASS AND O-LIFTING
C2B PU: 12 (w/#20 Vest)
Burpee: 10 (w/#20 Vest)
5 Rounds for time

GAMES WOD:
NOTE: IN ADDITION TO CLASS AND O-LIFTING
FSQ: 3
SJ: 3
EMOTM for 10 Minutes

Week 48

	SUNDAY 6/24	MONDAY 6/25	TUESDAY 6/26
WARM UP	**4 Rounds of** :15 Jumping Jack :15 Squat :15 MC :15 Jump Squat **Then** 30/20/30 w/bands PSN+PCL&J **Skill Set**	**4 Rounds of** :15 Jumping Jack :15 Squat :15 MC :15 Jump Squat **Then** Run/lunge 1x Run/butt kickers 1x Run/Straight Leg March 1x Run/power skips 1x Run/Spidey 1x Run/Cartwheel 1x Run/Toe Hold 1x Run/inchworm 1x **Then 4 Rounds of** :15 Plank :15 Superman :15 Side Plank /L :15 Side Plank /R **Then** 30/20/30 w/bands	**4 Rounds of** :15 Jumping Jack :15 Squat :15 MC :15 Jump Squat **Then** Run/lunge 1x Run/butt kickers 1x Run/Straight Leg March 1x Run/power skips 1x Run/Spidey 1x Run/Cartwheel 1x Run/Toe Hold 1x Run/inchworm 1x **Then 4 Rounds of** :15 Plank :15 Superman :15 Side Plank /L :15 Side Plank /R **Then** 30/20/30 w/bands
EQUIPMENT	SN BB: 70% of 1RM CL&J BB 70% of 1RM	Butcher 90/70	BB 185/135
WOD	PSN: 3 **EMOTM for 10 Min** **Rest 3:00** PCL and Jerk: 3 **EMOTM for 10 Min**	**A1** : Butcher HiPush **A2** : Butcher LoPush **A3** : Butcher HiPush **AMRAP: 15 Min**	FSQ: 10 Run: 200 **3 Rounds for time**
GAMES Phase III	All	**Active Rest**	All
SKILL/DEV WORK	TGU: 1R/1L x 10 T2B: 10 x 5 Sets Pistols: 10 x 5 Sets Hand Walk: 40ft **Then** Ring Hold Top Ring Hold Bottom **:20/:10 x 16 Alternating**	CHOICE	SN from Blocks (above knee): 2 x 10 Sets CL from Blocks (above knee): 2 x 10 Sets SJ from Blocks: 2 x 10 Sets **Load heavy, no time structure**
GAMES WOD All lifts @80% of 1RM	DL: 3 TH: 3 **EMOTM for 10 Min**		OHS: 3 BP: 3 **EMOTM for 10 Min**
ACCESSORY			GHD Sit Up: 12 GHD HB Ext: 12 **5 Rounds (Completion)**

WEDNESDAY 6/27	THURSDAY 6/28	FRIDAY 6/29	SATURDAY 6/30
4 Rounds of	**4 Rounds of**	**4 Rounds of**	Run/lunge 2x
:15 Jumping Jack	:15 Jumping Jack	:15 Jumping Jack	Run/butt kickers 2x
:15 Squat	:15 Squat	:15 Squat	Run/Straight Leg
:15 MC	:15 MC	:15 MC	March 2x
:15 Jump Squat	:15 Jump Squat	:15 Jump Squat	Run/power skips 2x
Then	**Then**	**Then**	Run/Spidey 2x
Run/lunge 1x	Run/lunge 1x	Run/lunge 1x	Run/Toes Hold 2x
Run/butt kickers 1x	Run/butt kickers 1x	Run/butt kickers 1x	Run/inchworm 2x
Run/Straight Leg March 1x	Run/Straight Leg March 1x	Run/Straight Leg March 1x	30/20/30 w/bands
Run/power skips 1x	Run/power skips 1x	Run/power skips 1x	
Run/Spidey 1x	Run/Spidey 1x	Run/Spidey 1x	
Run/Cartwheel 1x	Run/Cartwheel 1x	Run/Cartwheel 1x	
Run/Toe Hold 1x	Run/Toe Hold 1x	Run/Toe Hold 1x	
Run/inchworm 1x	Run/inchworm 1x	Run/inchworm 1x	
Then 4 Rounds of	**Then 4 Rounds of**	**Then 4 Rounds of**	
:15 Plank	:15 Plank	:15 Plank	
:15 Superman	:15 Superman	:15 Superman	
:15 Side Plank /L	:15 Side Plank /L	:15 Side Plank /L	
:15 Side Plank /R	:15 Side Plank /R	:15 Side Plank /R	
Then 30/20/30 w/bands	**Then** 30/20/30 w/bands	**Then** 30/20/30 w/bands	
Box 24/20		BB: 115/75	
Burpee Box Jump: 12	RPU: 5	Thruster: Max reps for :15	*Mary* or *Cindy*
Pull Up C2B: 12	T2B: 10	- Rest :45 - **for 15 Min**	**Games athletes**
4 Rounds for time	Wall Ball: 15		do *Mary*)
	AMRAP: 12 Min		
All + O-Lift	**Rest Day**	**All**	**All + O-Lift**
Rope Climb: 3		*Lift*	WOD #1
Run: 400			
3 Rounds for time			
		WOD/Skill/	WOD #2
			WOD #3

309

WEEK 48 -
SUN JUN 24 2012

PHASE III:

WARMUP:
4 Rounds of
:15 Jumping Jack
:15 Squat
:15 Mountain Climber
:15 Jump Squat
Then 30/20/30 w/bands
Skill Set for PSN+PCL&J

EQUIPMENT:
SN BB: 70% of 1RM;
CL&J BB 70% of 1RM

WOD:
PSN: 3 EMOTM for 10 Minutes
Then Rest 3:00
PCL and Jerk: 3 EMOTM for
10 Minutes

SKILL/DEV. WORK:
*NOTE: IN ADDITION TO
CLASS*
TGU: 1/1 x 10
T2B:
Pistol: 10 x 5 Sets
Hand Walk: 40ft
Then Ring Hold Top
Ring Hold Bottom
:20/10 x 16 Alternating

GAMES WOD:
*NOTE: IN ADDITION TO
CLASS*
DL: 3
TH: 3
EMOTM for 10 Minutes

WEEK 48 -
MON JUN 25 2012

PHASE III:

WARMUP:
4 Rounds of
:15 Jumping Jack
:15 Squat
:15 Mountain Climber
:15 Jump Squat
Then Run/lunge 1x
Run/butt kickers 1x
Run/Straight Leg March 1x
Run/power skips 1x
Run/Spidey 1x
Run/Cartwheel 1x
Run/Toe Hold 1x
Run/inchworm 1x
Then 4 Rounds of
:15 Plank
:15 Superman
:15 Side Plank - L
:15 Side Plank - R
Then 30/20/30 w/bands

EQUIPMENT:
Butcher 90/70

WOD:
P1: High Push
P2: Low Push
P3: High Push
AMRAP: 15 Minutes

GAMES: ACTIVE REST DAY

SKILL/DEV. WORK:
CHOICE

WEEK 48 -
TUE JUN 26 2012

PHASE III:

WARMUP:
4 Rounds of
:15 Jumping Jack
:15 Squat
:15 Mountain Climber
:15 Jump Squat
Then
Run/lunge 1x
Run/butt kickers 1x
Run/Straight Leg March 1x
Run/power skips 1x
Run/Spidey 1x
Run/Cartwheel 1x
Run/Toe Hold 1x
Run/inchworm 1x
Then 4 Rounds of
:15 Plank
:15 Superman
:15 Side Plank - L
:15 Side Plank - R
Then
30/20/30 w/bands

EQUIPMENT:
BB 185/135

WOD:
FSQ: 10
Run: 200
3 Rounds for time

SKILL/DEV. WORK:
NOTE: IN ADDITION TO CLASS
SN from Blocks
(Above Knee):
2 reps x 10 Sets

CL from Blocks
(Above Knee):
2 reps x 10 Sets

SJ from Blocks:
2 reps x 10 Sets
Load heavy -
No time structure

GAMES WOD:
NOTE: IN ADDITION TO CLASS
OHS: 3
BP: 3
EMOTM for 10 Minutes

ACCESSORY:
NOTE: IN ADDITION TO CLASS
GHD Sit Up: 12
GHD HB Ext: 12
5 Rounds (Completion)

311

WEEK 48 -
WED JUN 27 2012
PHASE III:
WARMUP:
4 Rounds of
:15 Jumping Jack
:15 Squat
:15 Mountain Climber
:15 Jump Squat
Then
Run/lunge 1x
Run/butt kickers 1x
Run/Straight Leg March 1x
Run/power skips 1x
Run/Spidey 1x
Run/Cartwheel 1x
Run/Toe Hold 1x
Run/inchworm 1x
Then 4 Rounds of
:15 Plank
:15 Superman
:15 Side Plank - L
:15 Side Plank - R
Then
30/20/30 w/bands
EQUIPMENT: Box 24/20
WOD:
Burpee Box Jump: 12
C2B Pull Up: 12
4 Rounds for time
SKILL/DEV. WORK:
NOTE: IN ADDITION TO
CLASS AND O-LIFTING
Rope Climb: 3
Run: 400
3 Rounds for time

WEEK 48 -
THU JUN 28 2012

PHASE III:

WARMUP:
4 Rounds of
:15 Jumping Jack
:15 Squat
:15 Mountain Climber
:15 Jump Squat
Then
Run/lunge 1x
Run/butt kickers 1x
Run/Straight Leg March 1x
Run/power skips 1x
Run/Spidey 1x
Run/Cartwheel 1x
Run/Toe Hold 1x
Run/inchworm 1x
Then 4 Rounds of
:15 Plank
:15 Superman
:15 Side Plank - L
:15 Side Plank - R
Then
30/20/30 w/bands

WOD:
RPU: 5
T2B: 10
Wall Ball: 15
AMRAP: 12 Minutes

GAMES: REST DAY

WEEK 48 - FRI JUN 29 2012

PHASE III:

WARMUP:
4 Rounds of
:15 Jumping Jack
:15 Squat
:15 Mountain Climber
:15 Jump Squat
Then
Run/lunge 1x
Run/butt kickers 1x
Run/Straight Leg March 1x
Run/power skips 1x
Run/Spidey 1x
Run/Cartwheel 1x
Run/Toe Hold 1x
Run/inchworm 1x
Then 4 Rounds of
:15 Plank
:15 Superman
:15 Side Plank - L
:15 Side Plank - R
Then
30/20/30 w/bands

EQUIPMENT:
BB: 115/75

WOD:
Thruster: Max Reps for :15 -
Rest :45 - for 15 Minutes

SKILL/DEV. WORK:
NOTE: IN ADDITION TO CLASS
Lift

GAMES WOD:
NOTE: IN ADDITION TO CLASS
WOD/Skill/Lift

WEEK 48 - SAT JUN 30 2012

PHASE III:

WARMUP:
Run/lunge 2x
Run/butt kickers 2x
Run/Straight Leg March 2x
Run/power skips 2x
Run/Spidey 2x
Run/Toes Hold 2x
Run/inchworm 2x
30/20/30 w/bands

WOD:
Mary or Cindy
(Games athletes do Mary)

SKILL/DEV. WORK:
NOTE: IN ADDITION TO CLASS AND O-LIFTING
WOD #1

GAMES WOD:
NOTE: IN ADDITION TO CLASS AND O-LIFTING
WOD #2

ACCESSORY:
NOTE: IN ADDITION TO CLASS AND O-LIFTING
WOD #3

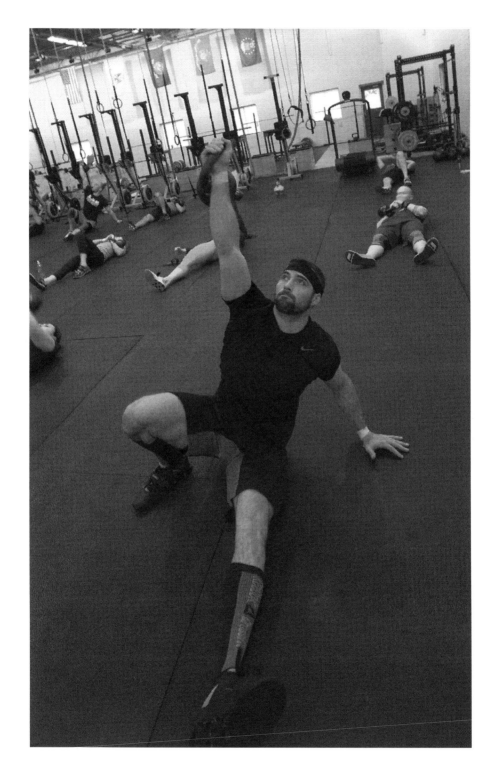

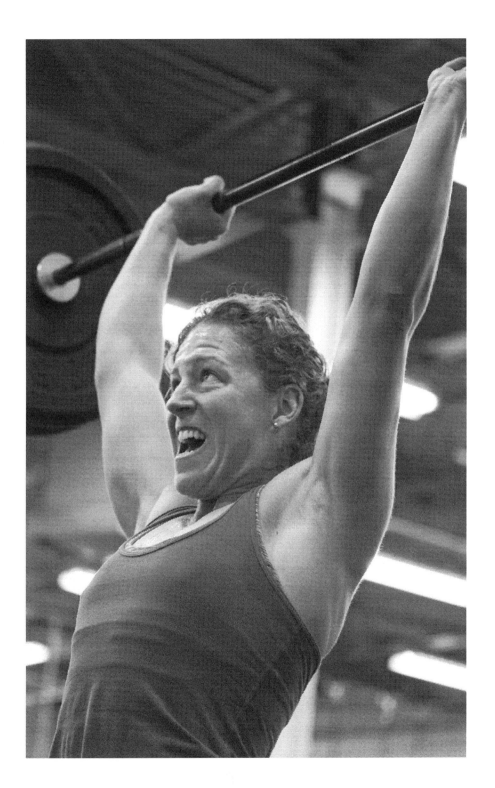

Week 49

	SUNDAY 7/1	MONDAY 7/2	TUESDAY 7/3
WARM UP	**4 Rounds of** :15 Jumping Jack :15 Squat :15 MC :15 Jump Squat **Then** 30/20/30 w/ bands	**4 Rounds of** :15 Jumping Jack :15 Squat :15 MC :15 Jump Squat **Then** Run/lunge 1x Run/butt kickers 1x Run/Straight Leg March 1x Run/power skips 1x Run/Spidey 1x Run/Cartwheel 1x Run/Toe Hold 1x Run/inchworm 1x **Then 4 Rounds of** :15 Plank :15 Superman :15 Side Plank /L :15 Side Plank /R **Then** 30/20/30 w/bands	**4 Rounds of** :15 Jumping Jack :15 Squat :15 MC :15 Jump Squat **Then** Run/lunge 1x Run/butt kickers 1x Run/Straight Leg March 1x Run/power skips 1x Run/Spidey 1x Run/Cartwheel 1x Run/Toe Hold 1x Run/inchworm 1x **Then 4 Rounds of** :15 Plank :15 Superman :15 Side Plank /L :15 Side Plank /R **Then** 30/20/30 w/ bands
EQUIPMENT	BB: 135/95	Dynamax: #20/14 Slam #30/20	BB 225/155 BB 95/65
WOD	SDLHP: 12 PP: 10 **5 Rounds for time**	Wall Ball: 12 Ball Slam: 10 **AMRAP: 5 Min - Rest 1:00 - 4 Rounds**	DL Thruster **21, 15, 9 for time**
GAMES Phase III	All	Active Rest	All
SKILL/DEV WORK		Swim: 25yds Burpee: 12 **AMRAP: 15 Min**	Ring Dip: 10 Pistols: 20 **4 Rounds for time**
GAMES WOD			BSQ: 2 x 5 Sets @90% of 1RM
ACCESSORY			HSPU: 12 GHD Sit Up: 12 **3 Rounds for time**

WEDNESDAY 7/4	THURSDAY 7/5	FRIDAY 7/6	SATURDAY 7/7
4 Rounds of	**4 Rounds of**	**4 Rounds of**	Run/lunge 2x
:15 Jumping Jack	:15 Jumping Jack	:15 Jumping Jack	Run/butt kickers 2x
:15 Squat	:15 Squat	:15 Squat	Run/Straight Leg
:15 MC	:15 MC	:15 MC	March 2x
:15 Jump Squat	:15 Jump Squat	:15 Jump Squat	Run/power skips 2x
Then	**Then**	**Then**	Run/Spidey 2x
Run/lunge 1x	Run/lunge 1x	Run/lunge 1x	Run/Toes Hold 2x
Run/butt kickers 1x	Run/butt kickers 1x	Run/butt kickers 1x	Run/inchworm 2x
Run/Straight Leg	Run/Straight Leg	Run/Straight Leg March 1x	30/20/30 w/bands
March 1x	March 1x	Run/power skips 1x	
Run/power skips 1x	Run/power skips 1x	Run/Spidey 1x	
Run/Spidey 1x	Run/Spidey 1x	Run/Cartwheel 1x	
Run/Cartwheel 1x	Run/Cartwheel 1x	Run/Toe Hold 1x	
Run/Toe Hold 1x	Run/Toe Hold 1x	Run/inchworm 1x	
Run/inchworm 1x	Run/inchworm 1x	**Then 4 Rounds of**	
Then 4 Rounds of	**Then 4 Rounds of**	:15 Plank	
:15 Plank	:15 Plank	:15 Superman	
:15 Superman	:15 Superman	:15 Side Plank /L	
:15 Side Plank /L	:15 Side Plank /L	:15 Side Plank /R	
:15 Side Plank /R	:15 Side Plank /R	**Then** 30/20/30 w/bands	
Then 30/20/30 w/ bands	**Then** 30/20/30 w/ bands		
Dynamax: #20/14 BB: #185/135	BB #135/95	BB 185/135	
Wall Ball: 50 PCL&J: 10 **3 Rounds for time**	Run: 400 BSQ: 30 **5 Rounds for time**	*Amanda* (Fat)	*DT*
All	**Rest Day**	**All**	**All**
		KBSN: 1R/1L x 12 T2B: 12 x 5 Sets MU: 7 x 5 Sets	
DL: 2 x 5 Sets @90% of 1RM		FSQ: 2 x 5 Sets @90% of 1RM	CL&J: 2 x 5 Sets @90% of 1RM
		SNBAL: 2 x 5 Sets @90% of 1RM HSN: 2 x 5 Sets @90% of 1RM	

317

WEEK 49 - SUN JUL 01 2012

PHASE III:

WARMUP:
4 Rounds of
:15 Jumping Jack
:15 Squat
:15 Mountain Climber
:15 Jump Squat
Then
30/20/30 w/bands

EQUIPMENT:
BB: 135/95

WOD:
SDLHP: 12
PP: 10
5 Rounds for time

NOTE:
TRANSITION TO PHASE IV
The final weeks of training focus on higher-intensity, lower-volume training. The strengthcomponents serve to maintain the gains achieved to date. The objective is to "rest" the athlete, yet at the same time, maintain an elevated "ready state."

WEEK 49 - MON JUL 02 2012

PHASE IV:

WARMUP:
4 Rounds of
:15 Jumping Jack
:15 Squat
:15 Mountain Climber
:15 Jump Squat
Then
Run/lunge 1x
Run/butt kickers 1x
Run/Straight Leg March 1x
Run/power skips 1x
Run/Spidey 1x
Run/Cartwheel 1x
Run/Toe Hold 1x
Run/inchworm 1x
Then 4 Rounds of
:15 Plank
:15 Superman
:15 Side Plank - L
:15 Side Plank - R
Then
30/20/30 w/bands

EQUIPMENT:
Dynamax: #20/14; Slam #30/20

WOD:
Wall Ball: 12
Ball Slam: 10
AMRAP: 5 Minutes -
Rest 1:00 - 4 Rounds

GAMES: ACTIVE REST DAY

SKILL/DEV. WORK:
Swim: 25yds
Burpee: 12
AMRAP: 15 Minutes

WEEK 49 - TUE JUL 03 2012

PHASE IV:

WARMUP:
4 Rounds of
:15 Jumping Jack
:15 Squat
:15 Mountain Climber
:15 Jump Squat
Then Run/lunge 1x
Run/butt kickers 1x
Run/Straight Leg March 1x
Run/power skips 1x
Run/Spidey 1x
Run/Cartwheel 1x
Run/Toe Hold 1x
Run/inchworm 1x
Then 4 Rounds of
:15 Plank
:15 Superman
:15 Side Plank - L
:15 Side Plank - R
Then 30/20/30 w/bands

EQUIPMENT:
BB 225/155; BB 95/65

WOD:
DLThruster
21, 15, 9 for time

SKILL/DEV. WORK:
NOTE: IN ADDITION TO CLASS
Ring Dip: 10
Pistol: 20
4 Rounds for time

GAMES WOD:
NOTE: IN ADDITION TO CLASS
BSQ: 2 reps x 5 Sets
@90% of 1RM

ACCESSORY:
NOTE: IN ADDITION TO CLASS
HSPU: 12
GHD Sit Up: 12
3 Rounds for time

WEEK 49 - WED JUL 04 2012

PHASE IV:

WARMUP:
4 Rounds of
:15 Jumping Jack
:15 Squat
:15 Mountain Climber
:15 Jump Squat
Then
Run/lunge 1x
Run/butt kickers 1x
Run/Straight Leg March 1x
Run/power skips 1x
Run/Spidey 1x
Run/Cartwheel 1x
Run/Toe Hold 1x
Run/inchworm 1x
Then 4 Rounds of
:15 Plank
:15 Superman
:15 Side Plank - L
:15 Side Plank - R
Then
30/20/30 w/bands

EQUIPMENT:
Dynamax: #20/14; BB: #185/135

WOD:
Wall Ball: 50
PCL&J: 10
3 Rounds for time

GAMES WOD:
NOTE: IN ADDITION TO CLASS
DL: 2 reps x 5 Sets
@90% of 1RM

WEEK 49 -
THU JUL 05 2012

PHASE IV:

WARMUP:
4 Rounds of
:15 Jumping Jack
:15 Squat
:15 Mountain Climber
:15 Jump Squat
Then
Run/lunge 1x
Run/butt kickers 1x
Run/Straight Leg March 1x
Run/power skips 1x
Run/Spidey 1x
Run/Cartwheel 1x
Run/Toe Hold 1x
Run/inchworm 1x
Then 4 Rounds of
:15 Plank
:15 Superman
:15 Side Plank - L
:15 Side Plank - R
Then
30/20/30 w/bands

EQUIPMENT:
BB #135/95

WOD:
Run: 400
BSQ: 30
5 Rounds for time

GAMES:
REST DAY

WEEK 49 -
FRI JUL 06 2012

PHASE IV:

WARMUP:
4 Rounds of
:15 Jumping Jack
:15 Squat
:15 Mountain Climber
:15 Jump Squat
Then
Run/lunge 1x
Run/butt kickers 1x
Run/Straight Leg March 1x
Run/power skips 1x
Run/Spidey 1x
Run/Cartwheel 1x
Run/Toe Hold 1x
Run/inchworm 1x
Then 4 Rounds of
:15 Plank
:15 Superman
:15 Side Plank - L
:15 Side Plank - R
Then
30/20/30 w/bands

EQUIPMENT:
BB 185/135

WOD:
Amanda (Fat)

CONTINUED>>>>>>>>>

WEEK 49 -
FRI JUL 06 2012
CONTINUED

SKILL/DEV. WORK:
NOTE: IN ADDITION TO CLASS
KBSN: 1/1 x 12
T2B: 12 reps x 5 Sets
MU: 7 Reps x 5 Sets

GAMES WOD:
NOTE: IN ADDITION TO CLASS
FSQ: 2 reps x 5 Sets
@90% of 1RM

ACCESSORY:
NOTE: IN ADDITION TO CLASS
SNBAL: 2 reps x 5 Sets
@90% of 1RM
HSN: 2 reps x 5 Sets
@90% of 1RM

WEEK 49 -
SAT JUL 07 2012

PHASE IV:

WARMUP:
Run/lunge 2x
Run/butt kickers 2x
Run/Straight Leg March 2x
Run/power skips 2x
Run/Spidey 2x
Run/Toes Hold 2x
Run/inchworm 2x
Then
30/20/30 w/bands

WOD:
DT

GAMES WOD:
NOTE: IN ADDITION TO CLASS
CL&J: 2 reps x 5 Sets
@90% of 1RM

Week 50

	SUNDAY 7/8	MONDAY 7/9	TUESDAY 7/10
WARM UP	**4 Rounds of** :15 Jumping Jack :15 Squat :15 MC :15 Jump Squat **Then** Run/lunge 1x Run/butt kickers 1x Run/Straight Leg March 1x Run/power skips 1x Run/Spidey 1x Run/Cartwheel 1x Run/Toe Hold 1x Run/inchworm 1x **Then 4 Rounds of** :15 Plank :15 Superman :15 Side Plank /L :15 Side Plank /R	30/20/30 w/Bands	Run: 400 30/20/30 w/Bands
EQUIPMENT	Box: 24/20	KB 24/16	BB 135/95
WOD	Run: 800 **Then** Ring Row: 12 Box Jump: 12 **4 Rounds for time**	American Swing: 20 Run: 200 **5 Rounds for time**	PCL&J: 30 **for time**
LIFTING/SKILL		BSQ 5-5-5-5-5 @80% of 1RM	FSQ 5-5-5-5-5 @80% of 1RM
GAMES Phase IV	Rest	Rest	TBA

NOTES

WEDNESDAY 7/11	THURSDAY 7/12	FRIDAY 7/13	SATURDAY 7/14
4 Rounds of	**4 Rounds of**	**4 Rounds of**	**4 Rounds of**
:15 Jumping Jack	:15 Jumping Jack	:15 Jumping Jack	:15 Jumping Jack
:15 Squat	:15 Squat	:15 Squat	:15 Squat
:15 MC	:15 MC	:15 MC	:15 MC
:15 Jump Squat	:15 Jump Squat	:15 Jump Squat	:15 Jump Squat
		Then	**Then**
		Run/lunge 1x	Run/lunge 1x
		Run/butt kickers 1x	Run/butt kickers 1x
		Run/Straight Leg March 1x	Run/Straight Leg March 1x
		Run/power skips 1x	Run/power skips 1x
		Run/Spidey 1x	Run/Spidey 1x
		Run/Cartwheel 1x	Run/Cartwheel 1x
		Run/Toe Hold 1x	Run/Toe Hold 1x
		Run/inchworm 1x	Run/inchworm 1x
		Then 4 Rounds of	**Then 4 Rounds of**
		:15 Plank	:15 Plank
		:15 Superman	:15 Superman
		:15 Side Plank /L	:15 Side Plank /L
		:15 Side Plank /R	:15 Side Plank /R
		Then 30/20/30 w/Bands	
BB: 95/65	BB 125/75	Sandbag #70/50 Slammer 30/20	You
4 Rounds of	PSN: 12	**A1** : Sandbag Run: 50yds	*Angie*
Push Press: 12	Pull Up: 10	**A2** : Push Up (Score)	
Dip: 12	**3 Rounds for time**	**A3** : Ball Slam (Score)	
Run: 200		**AMRAP: 12 Min**	
DL 5-5-5-5-5 @80% of 1RM	OHS 5-5-5-5-5 **E3M** @80% of 1RM		
TBA	**Active Rest**	**Rest**	**Class Only**

NOTES

_____

_____

_____

_____

WEEK 50 - SUN JUL 08 2012

PHASE IV:

WARMUP:
4 Rounds of
:15 Jumping Jack
:15 Squat
:15 Mountain Climber
:15 Jump Squat
Then
Run/lunge 1x
Run/butt kickers 1x
Run/Straight Leg March 1x
Run/power skips 1x
Run/Spidey 1x
Run/Cartwheel 1x
Run/Toe Hold 1x
Run/inchworm 1x
Then 4 Rounds of
:15 Plank
:15 Superman
:15 Side Plank - L
:15 Side Plank - R

EQUIPMENT:
Box: 24/20

WOD:
Run: 800
Then
Ring Row: 12
Box Jump: 12
4 Rounds for time

GAMES:
REST DAY

WEEK 50 - MON JUL 09 2012

PHASE IV:

WARMUP:
30/20/30 w/Bands

EQUIPMENT:
KB 24/16

WOD:
American Swing: 20
Run: 200
5 Rounds for time

LIFTING/SKILL DEV:
BSQ 5-5-5-5-5 E3M

GAMES:
REST DAY

WEEK 50 -
TUE JUL 10 2012

PHASE IV:

WARMUP:
Run: 400
30/20/30 w/Bands

EQUIPMENT:
BB 135/95

WOD:
PCL&J: 30 for time

LIFTING/SKILL DEV:
FSQ 5-5-5-5-5 E3M

GAMES:
TBA

WEEK 50 -
WED JUL 11 2012

PHASE IV:

WARMUP:
4 Rounds of
:15 Jumping Jack
:15 Squat
:15 Mountain Climber
:15 Jump Squat

EQUIPMENT:
BB: 95/65

WOD:
4 Rounds of
Push Press: 12
Dip: 12
Run: 200

LIFTING/SKILL DEV:
DL 5-5-5-5-5 E3M

GAMES: T
BA

WEEK 50 - THU JUL 12 2012

PHASE IV:

WARMUP:
4 Rounds of
:15 Jumping Jack
:15 Squat
:15 Mountain Climber
:15 Jump Squat

EQUIPMENT:
BB 125/75

WOD:
PSN: 12
Pull Up: 10
3 Rounds for time

LIFTING/SKILL DEV:
OHS 5-5-5-5-5 E3M

GAMES:
ACTIVE REST DAY

WEEK 50 - FRI JUL 13 2012

PHASE IV:

WARMUP:
4 Rounds of
:15 Jumping Jack
:15 Squat
:15 Mountain Climber
:15 Jump Squat
Then
Run/lunge 1x
Run/butt kickers 1x
Run/Straight Leg March 1x
Run/power skips 1x
Run/Spidey 1x
Run/Cartwheel 1x
Run/Toe Hold 1x
Run/inchworm 1x
Then 4 Rounds of
:15 Plank
:15 Superman
:15 Side Plank - L
:15 Side Plank - R
Then
30/20/30 w/Bands

EQUIPMENT:
Sandbag #70/50;
Slammer 30/20

WOD:
P1: Sandbag Run: 50yds
P2: Push Up (Score)
P3: Ball Slam (Score)
AMRAP: 12 Minutes

GAMES: REST DAY

WEEK 50 -
SAT JUL 14 2012

PHASE IV:

WARMUP:
4 Rounds of
:15 Jumping Jack
:15 Squat
:15 Mountain Climber
:15 Jump Squat
Then
Run/lunge 1x
Run/butt kickers 1x
Run/Straight Leg March 1x
Run/power skips 1x
Run/Spidey 1x
Run/Cartwheel 1x
Run/Toe Hold 1x
Run/inchworm 1x
Then 4 Rounds of
:15 Plank
:15 Superman
:15 Side Plank - L
:15 Side Plank - R

EQUIPMENT:
You

WOD:
Angie

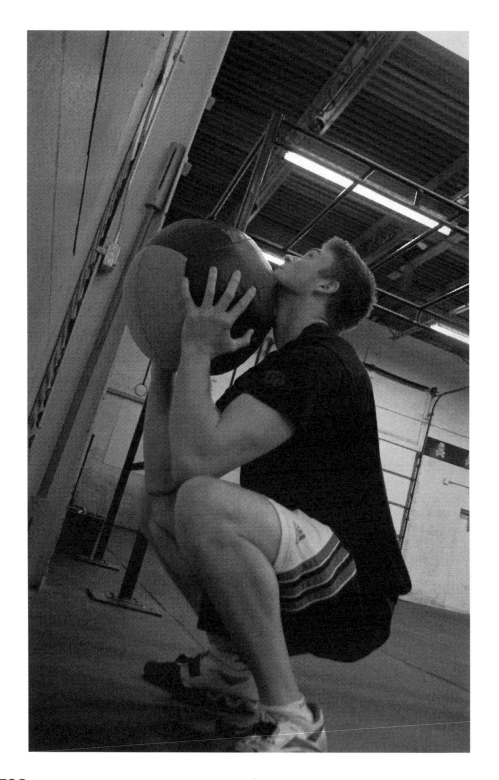

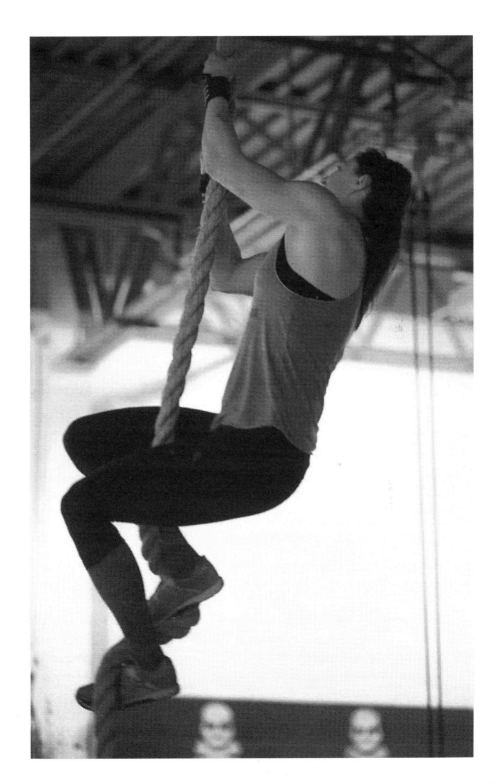

Outro

CrossFit is a community, and we need your feedback to help us make the next version better! We value your comments and your reviews.

Please take the time to write a quick review on Amazon, or email to questions@hyperfitusa.com with comments or questions.

This book is a slice of history. It is not our current regimen. Coaching and programming develop over time. There were many great lessons learned from the 2012 Games season. We programmed them into our training, which we constantly improve through further tweaks and changes.

Because training evolves constantly, it's beneficial to keep up with the current equipment and techniques.

For information about upcoming camps and personal training, please email to training@hyperfitusa.com

Drop by our webpage at www.hyperfitusa.com to see what's happening at our gym.

Or visit our Facebook page:
https://www.facebook.com/pages/HyperFit-USA-CrossFit-Ann-Arbor/46194210949

Glossary

Information on named and benchmark workouts (**Elizabeth, Murph, Angie, The Chief, Cindy**, etc.) and special occasions (**Olympic Lifting, Organized Mobility, Instructor Games**, etc.) can be found at www.crossfit.com, on the CrossFit website.

21-15-9 or **21, 15, 9** :: 21, then 15, then 9 reps of each move :: *Miscellaneous*

30/20/30 :: 30 Squats, 20 Shoulder Rollovers, 30 Overhead Squats with PVC pipe :: *WarmUp/CoolDown Moves*

5 Min Left :: *WarmUp/CoolDown Moves*

5 Min Right :: *WarmUp/CoolDown Moves*

75% of Max :: 75% of your Personal Record :: *Miscellaneous*

ABMat :: AbMat Sit-Up :: *WarmUp/CoolDown Moves*

ABMat :: AbMat Sit-Up :: *WOD/Games Training Moves*

AMRAP :: As Many Rounds As Possible :: *Miscellaneous*

Ankles Up :: *WarmUp/CoolDown Moves*

AS :: American KB Swing :: *WOD/Games Training Moves*

AS :: Air Squat :: *WarmUp/CoolDown Moves*

Back extensions :: *WOD/Games Training Moves*

BB :: Barbell :: *Equipment*

Bearcrawl :: *WarmUp/CoolDown Moves*

BJ :: Box Jump :: *WOD/Games Training Moves*

Blocks :: *Equipment*

Box :: Sturdy platform to jump on, 20 or 30 inches high :: *Equipment*

BSQ :: Back Squat :: *WOD/Games Training Moves*

Burpee :: Burpee :: *WOD/Games Training Moves*

Butcher Hi/Butcher Low :: Butcher push sled with High/Low push bars :: *Equipment*

BW or BWT :: Body weight :: *Miscellaneous*

C2 :: Concept 2 Rowing machine :: *Equipment*

Cartwheels :: *WarmUp/CoolDown Moves*

CBPU :: Chest to Bar pull-up :: *WOD/Games Training Moves*

CL :: Clean :: *WOD/Games Training Moves*

CL&J :: Clean And Jerk :: *WOD/Games Training Moves*

Cluster :: Clean into a thruster :: *WOD/Games Training Moves*

Crabwalk :: *WarmUp/CoolDown Moves*

Cross Over Push-Up :: Cross Over Push-Up(Moving across a KB) :: *WOD/Games Training Moves*

DB :: Dumbbell :: *Equipment*

DB High Pull :: Dumbbell High Pull :: *WOD/Games Training Moves*

DB squat Clean :: Dumbbell Squat Clean :: *WOD/Games Training Moves*

DBHSN :: Dumbbell Hang Snatch :: *WOD/Games Training Moves*

DHPU :: Dead Hang Pull-Up :: *WOD/Games Training Moves*

Dip :: Dips :: *WOD/Games Training Moves*

DL :: Deadlift :: *WOD/Games Training Moves*

DSN :: Drop Snatch :: *WOD/Games Training Moves*

DU :: Double Under :: *WOD/Games Training Moves*

E3M :: Every 3 Min :: *Miscellaneous*

EMOTM :: Every Minute On The Minute :: *Miscellaneous*

Farmers walk :: *WOD/Games Training Moves*

FGB :: Fight Gone Bad :: *WOD/Games Training Moves*

Flutter kicks :: *WarmUp/CoolDown Moves*

FR :: Floor Row :: *WOD/Games Training Moves*

FSQ :: Front Squat :: *WOD/Games Training Moves*

GHD :: Glute Hamstring Developer :: *WOD/Games Training Moves*

GHD :: Glute Hamstring Developer :: *Equipment*

GHD Back Extension :: *WOD/Games Training Moves*

GHD Hip and Back Extension :: *WOD/Games Training Moves*

GHD Sit-Up :: *WOD/Games Training Moves*

Good Morning :: Hamstring Exercise :: *WOD/Games Training Moves*

H2H swing :: Hand to Hand KB Swing :: *WOD/Games Training Moves*

Hand walk :: Walk on hands :: *WOD/Games Training Moves*

Handle Carry :: Strong Man Handle Walk :: *WOD/Games Training Moves*

Heel Kicks :: *WarmUp/CoolDown Moves*

HPCL :: Hang Power Clean :: *WOD/Games Training Moves*

HRPU :: Hand Release Push-Up :: *WOD/Games Training Moves*

HRPU :: Hand Release Push-Up :: *WarmUp/CoolDown Moves*

HSNBAL :: Heave Snatch Balance :: *WOD/Games Training Moves*

HSPU :: Hand Stand Push-Up :: *WOD/Games Training Moves*

Inch Worm :: *WarmUp/CoolDown Moves*

J :: Jerk (Shoulder to Overhead) :: *WOD/Games Training Moves*

JJ :: Jumping Jack :: *WarmUp/CoolDown Moves*

Jog :: 50% Speed (approximately) :: *WOD/Games Training Moves*

JS :: Jump Squat :: *WarmUp/CoolDown Moves*

JSQT :: Jump Squat :: *WOD/Games Training Moves*

Jumping :: Plyometrics :: *WOD/Games Training Moves*

K2E :: Knees to elbows, hanging from bar :: *WOD/Games Training Moves*

KB :: Kettlebell :: *Equipment*

KBSN :: Kettlebell Snatch :: *WOD/Games Training Moves*

Kettlebell Rack Walk :: *WOD/Games Training Moves*

L-Sit :: L-sit :: *WOD/Games Training Moves*

Ladder :: Do 1 rep, then 2 reps, then 3, up to whatever you can :: *Miscellaneous*

Load Heavy :: Go as heavy as possible :: *Miscellaneous*

Low Box :: 6-inch Box :: *WOD/Games Training Moves*

Low Box :: Step or low box, 6 or 8 inches high :: *Equipment*

Lunge :: *WarmUp/CoolDown Moves*

Max Reps :: as many reps as you can in the allotted time :: *Miscellaneous*

MBCL :: Med Ball Clean :: *WOD/Games Training Moves*

MC :: Mountain Climber :: *WOD/Games Training Moves*

MC :: Mountain Climbers :: *WarmUp/CoolDown Moves*

Mobility :: Mobility WOD :: *Miscellaneous*

MSCL :: Muscle Clean :: *WOD/Games Training Moves*

MSSN :: Muscle Snatch :: *WOD/Games Training Moves*

MU :: Muscle Up :: *WOD/Games Training Moves*

OHS :: Overhead Squat :: *WOD/Games Training Moves*

PCL :: Power Clean :: *WOD/Games Training Moves*

PCL&J :: Power Clean and Jerk :: *WOD/Games Training Moves*

Pistol :: Pistol Squats :: *WOD/Games Training Moves*

PJ :: Push Jerk :: *WOD/Games Training Moves*

Plank Hold :: *WarmUp/CoolDown Moves*

Power Skip :: *WarmUp/CoolDown Moves*

PP :: Push Press :: *WOD/Games Training Moves*

PR :: Personal Record :: *Miscellaneous*

Press :: Barbell Press :: *WOD/Games Training Moves*

Prison Rules :: Just get it up there any way you can! :: *Miscellaneous*

Pro Agility :: *WarmUp/CoolDown Moves*

PSN :: Power Snatch :: *WOD/Games Training Moves*

PU :: Push-Up :: *WOD/Games Training Moves*

PU :: Pull-Up - can also mean Push-Up! :: *WOD/Games Training Moves*

PU (Weighted) :: Weighted Pull-Up :: *WOD/Games Training Moves*

Rack :: Squat Rack :: *Equipment*

RDL :: Romanian Deadlift :: *WOD/Games Training Moves*

Rep :: Repetition; one performance of an exercise :: *Miscellaneous*

Reverse Hyper :: Reverse Hyperextensions - Machine :: *WOD/Games Training Moves*

Reverse ladder :: 10 reps, then 9,8,7,6,5,4,3,2,1 :: *Miscellaneous*

Ring Dip :: Ring Dips :: *WOD/Games Training Moves*

Ring Row :: Ring Row :: *WOD/Games Training Moves*

Rings :: Gymnastic Rings :: *Equipment*

RM :: Rep Max :: *Miscellaneous*

Roll :: To roll out :: *Miscellaneous*

Roll and recovery :: *WarmUp/CoolDown Moves*

Roller :: Hard foam roller to work muscle tension :: *Equipment*

ROM :: Range of Motion :: *Miscellaneous*

Rope Climb :: Rope Climb :: *WOD/Games Training Moves*

ROW :: Using Concept 2 Rowing machine :: *WOD/Games Training Moves*

RPU :: Ring Push-Ups :: *WOD/Games Training Moves*

RS :: Russian Swing :: *WOD/Games Training Moves*

Run :: 80% Speed (approximately) :: *WOD/Games Training Moves*

Run :: *WarmUp/CoolDown Moves*

Rx'd :: As prescribed; as written, no adjustments :: *Miscellaneous*

Sandbag :: *Equipment*

Sandbag run :: *WOD/Games Training Moves*

SDL :: Sumo Deadlift :: *WOD/Games Training Moves*

SDLHP :: Sumo Deadlift High Pull :: *WOD/Games Training Moves*

Side Plank :: *WarmUp/CoolDown Moves*

SJ :: Split Jerk :: *WOD/Games Training Moves*

Slam :: Ball Slam :: *WOD/Games Training Moves*

Slammer :: Ball Slam Ball :: *Equipment*

Sled :: Sled with weight to push :: *Equipment*

Sled Drag :: Sled Drag :: *WOD/Games Training Moves*

SN :: Snatch :: *WOD/Games Training Moves*

SNBAL :: Snatch Balance :: *WOD/Games Training Moves*

SP :: Sostz Press :: *WOD/Games Training Moves*

Spiderman :: *WarmUp/CoolDown Moves*

Split Squat :: *WarmUp/CoolDown Moves*

Sprint :: 100% Speed :: *WOD/Games Training Moves*

SQSN :: Full Squat Snatch :: *WOD/Games Training Moves*

SQT :: Air Squat :: *WOD/Games Training Moves*

Steps :: Number of Lunge Steps :: *WOD/Games Training Moves*

Stove Pipe :: Static KB hold - Rack Position :: *WOD/Games Training Moves*

Straight Leg March :: *WarmUp/CoolDown Moves*

SU :: Sit-Up :: *WOD/Games Training Moves*

Superman :: *WarmUp/CoolDown Moves*

Swing :: Kettlebell Swing (Default is Russian) :: *WOD/Games Training Moves*

T2B :: Toes To Bar :: *WOD/Games Training Moves*

Tabata :20/:10 :: Move for 20 seconds, rest for 10 seconds; usually 8 rounds of first move, then 1 min rest, then 8 rounds of next move :: *Miscellaneous*

TGU :: Turkish Get Up :: *WOD/Games Training Moves*

TH :: Thruster :: *WOD/Games Training Moves*

Up and down the ladder :: 1 rep, then 2,3,4,5,4,3,2,1 :: *Miscellaneous*

Vest :: Weighted vest :: *Equipment*

Waiter's Walk :: *WOD/Games Training Moves*

Walking Lunge :: Walking Lunges - High Carry :: *WOD/Games Training Moves*

Walking Lunge :: *WarmUp/CoolDown Moves*

Wall Walk :: *WOD/Games Training Moves*

WB :: Wall Ball :: *WOD/Games Training Moves*

WB :: Wall Ball/Dynamax Ball :: *Equipment*

Windmill :: *WOD/Games Training Moves*

WOD :: Workout of the day :: *Miscellaneous*

Woodway :: Woodway treadmill :: *Equipment*

ZS :: Zercher Squat :: *WOD/Games Training Moves*

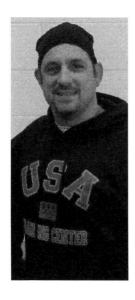

ABOUT THE AUTHOR:

Douglas Chapman coaches top CrossFit competitors Andrea Ager, Jennifer Smith, Neal Maddox, and many others. He trained Julie Foucher to win the title of The 2nd Fittest Woman on Earth in the 2012 CrossFit Games; she will be training with Doug again for the 2014 Games.

Doug is the owner of HyperFit USA, one of CrossFit's 20 original affiliates (the 13th such facility to embrace the sport); he has been coaching for over 20 years.
DChap (as he is also known) was nicknamed "The Wizard of WODs" by some of his athletes, for his unique talent of creating highly effective, varied, progressive and cohesive CrossFit programming. Doug is an alumnus of Eastern Michigan University and the US Navy, and holds 20 fitness certifications covering a wide range of disciplines.

Made in the USA
Lexington, KY
13 March 2014